Mental Health and Human Rights in Palestine

Mental Health and Human Rights in Palestine

The Life of Gaza's Pioneering Psychiatrist Dr Eyad Sarraj

by
Wasseem El Sarraj

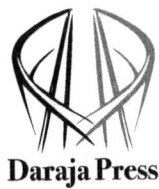

Daraja Press

Published by
Daraja Press
https://darajapress.com

In association with
Zand Graphics Ltd (Kenya)
https://zandgraphics.com

© 2022 Wasseem El Sarraj
All rights reserved

ISBN 9781990263378

Cover design: Kate McDonnell

Library and Archives Canada Cataloguing in Publication

Title: Mental health and human rights in Palestine : the life of Gaza's pioneering psychiatrist Dr Eyad Sarraj / Wasseem El Sarraj.
Names: El Sarraj, Wasseem, author.
Description: Includes bibliographical references.
Identifiers: Canadiana (print) 20220159270 | Canadiana (ebook) 20220159297 | ISBN 9781990263378 (softcover) | ISBN 9781990263385 (ebook)
Subjects: LCSH: Sarraj, Eyad. | LCSH: Psychiatrists—Gaza Strip—Gaza—Biography. | LCGFT: Biographies.
Classification: LCC RC438.6 .E4 2022 | DDC 616.89/14092—dc23

For Ali and Samir

*Knowledge builds houses from broken stones
Ignorance destroys once glorious houses.*
—Arabic Poem, from Abu Sitta's memoir:
Mapping My Return: A Palestinian Memoir

CONTENTS

Foreword by Ruchama Marton, MD — xi
Preface — xv
Prologue — xviii

1. Empires and Tribes — 1
2. The British — 5
3. The *Nakba* — 16
4. Egypt: Collective Joy — 28
5. Returning to Gaza — 35
6. London — 41
7. The Clinician and the Activist — 48
8. The Gaza Community Mental Healthcare Programme — 60
9. 'If you have the gun, you have the rights' — 70
10. War on Gaza — 80
11. A talent for hope — 85
12. The rationality of revolt — 95
Epilogue — 101

Afterword by Yasser Abu Jamei, Director of the GCMHP — 107

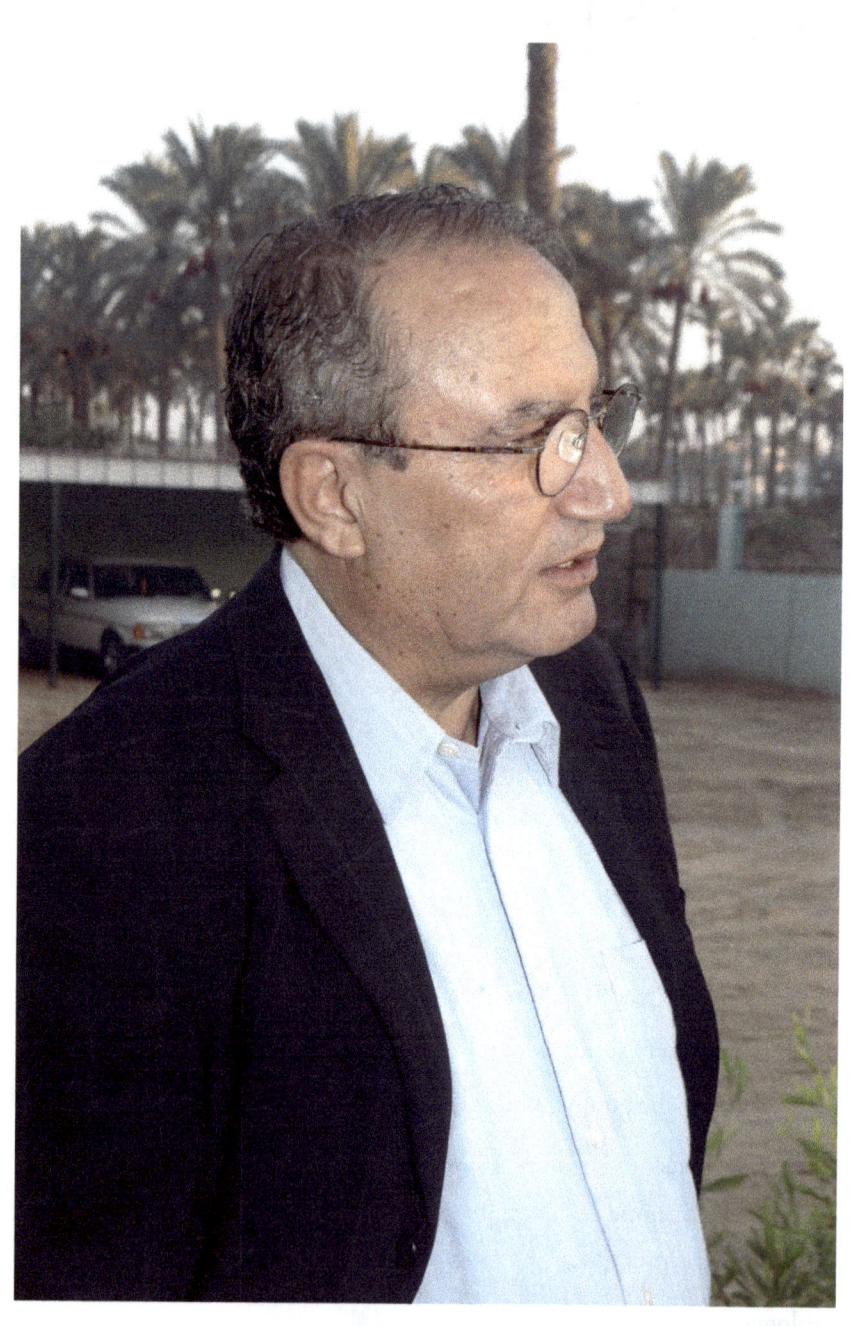

Eyad Sarraj, 1944 – 2013

FOREWORD BY RUCHAMA MARTON, MD

The book gives a socio-political background necessary for the reader to understand the complicated situations and conditions, especially in the Palestinian and Israeli long and bloody conflict that was the framework for Eyad's life, thinking, and professional and political activity.

As a reader, the passionate way Wasseem describes his father is touching and gives an excellent picture of the person that Eyad was.

I met Eyad in Gaza at the very beginning of the first Intifada.

Gaza, January 1988, it was freezing. The streets were deserted. Streets, passages of mud and rainwater mixed with sewage water which had no efficient drainage. Kids, lips blue from the cold, allowed our white van to pass despite the general strike declared in Gaza. It was a total strike: all the stores were closed, and no cars were on the road.

The van arrived at Shifa Hospital. It was icy in the hospital as well. Nevertheless, the place was packed with people. All the beds were filled with young people injured from beatings or shooting by Israeli soldiers.

There we, an Israeli group of doctors, met Dr Eyad Sarraj. He was a tall man with curly hair and a charming smile. He escorted us, explaining the harsh sights of the wounded young people and the neglect and filth in Shifa's governmental hospital in a soft voice. After a long day in the hospital, Eyad invited us, the Israeli doctors' delegation, to his private home in the Rimal neighbourhood. The conversation was conducted in English. In the beginning, it was hard for us. The sight of the wounded and the miserable conditions at the hospital caused most the Israelis to be defensive. "We are not an investigative committee," said one of the Israeli doctors. However, Eyad understood the complex situation and softened the Israeli defensive aggression. After an hour and a half at his home, the group's mood became easy and cooperative. It was Eyad who led the process and the change in our group. For Eyad and me, it was the beginning of a long friendship.

Two months later, in Tel Aviv, the founding conference for the Association of Israeli and Palestinian Physicians for Human Rights was held. The theatre was packed with Israeli physicians, physicians from the Gaza Strip, East Jerusalem, the West Bank, and the Golan Heights. Eyad was on stage translating from Arabic to English and vice versa. Someone from the Golan Height presented himself in Arabic: 'I am a doctor from occupied southern Syria.' Eyad said in English: 'This is a comrade from the Golan Heights'. A man shouted from the hall's back row: 'That's a lie! I understand Arabic. He said that he is from southern Syria! You're being deceived here. This meeting should be dissolved!' There was a commotion in the hall, and the meeting was about to blow up. Eyad took the microphone and said in a loud voice: 'Please sit down. I made a mistake. I didn't understand the comrade's words well enough. I'll translate again, and this time, precisely.' The explosion was avoided.

Eyad continued: 'I'm a Palestinian physician from Gaza. I'm proud to be part of the establishment of this physician's organization for human rights. I call all of you to take part in it.'

This intervention was typical for Eyad, as we can learn from Wasseem's book. He found the right way to do things with his sensitivity and problem-solving skills.

Thank you, Eyad.

We met many times during the following years, in Tel Aviv, at conferences abroad, but mainly in Gaza.

The Israeli security forces perceived Eyad as dangerous. Many Palestinians who believed in a non-violent struggle toward peace with Israelis found themselves in jail. I received a telephone call from the Gaza health headquarters officer one day. They asked for a meeting as soon as possible. During the meeting, they asked me: 'What do you know about Dr Eyad al-Sarraj? Do not think that you're the only Israeli woman who has contact with Eyad. He has lots of Israeli women. I want to warn you for your own good.' I ended the meeting immediately. The next day, Eyad was arrested by the army and deported from Gaza.

He was in London for two and a half years. He collected money and returned to Gaza, able to fulfil his dream of establishing a mental healthcare centre in Gaza (1992). This was not a simple thing to do in a community where there was no respect for mental health, no infrastructure, and no professional personnel. Nevertheless, Eyad created something big out of nothing.

Eyad and I met at many conferences, where it was possible to talk about many personal and political issues. We discovered that we had both started out in medicine as paediatricians, and afterwards, we had chosen to specialize in psychiatry, which we both were happy about.

Eyad didn't belong to any political party in Gaza; no one else in Gaza had taken that stand. As a person with an independent spirit and a leader's character, he fought for human rights, particularly for the rights of Palestinians. He disagreed with the general opinion – first, we'll fight the Occupation, and only then, we'll fight for the integrity of people at home. He laughed when I told him that he spoke like a feminist. 'Me? I grew up with a mother and several sisters. It was forbidden for me to enter the kitchen and take a glass of water for myself. My mother always said that I had to be served.' True, I agreed with him; you demand and receive service. However, there is a similarity: the radical feminists never agreed with the prevailing opinion that first we attain social equality and then we can fight for women's rights. That is exactly what you say about your struggle for incorruptibility in the Palestinian Authority. Eyad agreed and said with a big smile: 'You'll make a great feminist out of me yet.'

The Palestinian Authority didn't like his political independence and opinions. As a result, Eyad was arrested twice during the time of Chairman Yasser Arafat in 1995-6. He spent long days in solitary confinement, in harsh conditions of imprisonment, where he suffered greatly as he wasn't used to such conditions. Above all, he suffered from the humiliation of his imprisonment. Eyad was a proud person who couldn't withstand such an attitude. Being imprisoned by his own people depressed him. It took a long time and many conversations for him to return to himself.

In the meantime, the Gaza Community Mental Health Care Programme (GCMHP) progressed and functioned as a centre. Eyad was particularly concerned for children and youth. He dealt with their difficult emotional situation. The traditional family structure had been destroyed right before their eyes: the father having lost his place in the family, either through being beaten and humiliated by Israeli soldiers in front of the family or by the humiliation of forced unemployment.

In this book, Wasseem discusses Eyad's role as a father figure in the Gaza community, especially in GCMHP.

Eyad fought for women's rights in Gaza and created a special therapeutic framework for them. That was not an easy task in a traditional society where there was an accelerated process of turning to religion.

Eyad published articles about his psychological understanding of children and youth in the Palestinian community in Gaza. His articles merited much international attention.

All along our shared route, Eyad was an inseparable part of the struggle against torture. His voice was heard in conferences against torture throughout the world. We often appeared as a team – the Israeli and the Palestinian struggling together against torture, administrative detention and prison conditions. Eyad also didn't hesitate to criticize the Palestinian Authority regarding arrests and torture. In the Gaza Center for Mental Health, he trained special staff who treated prisoners and those who had been tortured.

In 2008, the Israeli army bombed the GCMHP building. The destruction was immense, and Eyad found it difficult to deal with it. I met him sometime after the bombing. He looked awful. He was sick. And then, the blood disease he had suffered from was revealed. Eyad had spent many years in his struggle against malignant leukaemia, from which he eventually died in a hospital in Israel.

One can say that Eyad was born in Palestine, died in Israel but lived in Gaza.

As Wasseem writes: Gaza's pain was Eyad's pain.

Ruchama Marton, MD is an Israeli psychotherapist, psychiatrist, feminist, and founder of Physicians for Human Rights-Israel

PREFACE

> *If you think about it seriously, all the questions about the soul and the immortality of the soul and paradise and hell are at the bottom only a way of seeing this very simple fact that every action of ours is passed on to others according to its value, of good or evil, it passes from father to son, from one generation to the next, in a perpetual movement.* — Gramsci

'God bless your wandering soul,' my father, Eyad Sarraj, wrote to me in 2008. He was replying to me after learning I was struggling to figure out my path in life. It was typically poetic of him. It conveyed an appreciation for my emotional world and left open any judgment on the right path forward. Only now, in 2021, reading interviews with his friends, I see this thread of his character that carried through in his relationships.

Hasan Ziada, a colleague from the Gaza Community Mental Health Program (GCMHP), the mental health clinic Eyad founded, remarks that Eyad was like this, always seeking to encourage, in a warm way, but not overpowering or judgmental. It made him a father figure for many in Palestine and his colleagues at GCMHP. In addition, he was incredibly intuitive, picking up on moods and feelings in his own community. This intuition, and his moral principles, combined with being an excellent communicator, helped make him an influential figure in Gaza and a renowned global advocate for Palestinian rights.

Eyad tried many times to write his memoir with many different people. Finally, in 2016, I took on the responsibility to finish what he started, and I crowdfunded to write his biography. The book would pay tribute to his legacy as a mental health pioneer in Gaza and as a human rights campaigner. At the time, it seemed like a straightforward idea. What I had not fully processed was how emotionally challenging it would be. Nor had I realised how much I would struggle with the weight of expectation and responsibility. Eventually, after having time to process grief and deal with the trauma of war, I found my voice. In fact, the writing, and researching, the process became a source of healing.

The following is a biography of my father's life. It is also a history of Palestine with a focus on Gaza. My father's life was so intertwined with Palestine that his choices and reactions reflect many of the major historical moments of the last 70 years. The book is an effort to understand how the forces around him impacted his life, how he took control of what he could, and what he could achieve in an intractable situation. The book is also interspersed with my own reflections, derived – in part – from being the son of a Palestinian. It is a perspective that offers a way of seeing Palestine through my British identity. Observations are also based on living and working in Gaza for several years. During this period, I experienced Israel's 2012 war on Gaza: a war that left me – and many others – with traumatic wounds.

In this context, I imagined various readers. Firstly, I hope that this book is appreciated by people who knew, loved, and admired Eyad. I know he had many friends and colleagues who considered him an important part of their lives. Whether it was as someone, they could talk to, work with, or as someone who inspired them to do better in the world. I hope I have captured this spirit that many found so edifying. Secondly, the book hopefully serves as a modest introduction to Palestine. I have relied on the careful and humbling work of Palestinian historians such as Rashid Khalidi. There is a vast and rich literature on Palestine, and many themes in the book, such as peace talks, human rights, civil society and historical trauma, have been explored elsewhere in much greater depth. For readers interested in learning more about these issues, I have compiled a reading list found at the back of the book.

Lastly, as a young bi-racial (half Palestinian/half English) man growing up in Western Europe, issues of identity and belonging crop up regularly. Dominant cultural and national discourses often leave out the stories of Palestinians. This can be confusing as you try to make sense of the world about your Palestinian identity. This can be made more difficult without the proximity to your Palestinian family. As a result, many children in the Palestinian diaspora don't speak Arabic; and don't, or can't, visit Palestine. I hope my story, my father's story, provides some help in making sense of their experiences.

The book would not have been possible without the support of those who donated. You have been kind, patient, and thoughtful, and that space and understanding have finally allowed this book to be completed. I also would like to thank Paul Aaron, Tom Hill, Arthur Neslen, John Van Eenwyk, David Henley, Henrik Pelling and Sara Roy. Aside from knowing and loving, Eyad, they have also written about Eyad and/or conducted interviews with either Eyad or his friends and colleagues. I also want to give a special thanks to Liz Berger, Colin Green, Gerri Haynes, Brian Barber, Nancy Murray, Mahmoud Sharafi, Marwan Diab, Daragh Murray, and Michael Morse for their friendship and mentorship. And lastly, I want to thank Hiba, my wife, who – during a challenging time – not only provided wise edits but has been endlessly encouraging and understanding.

I would like to also pay tribute to Eyad's friends and colleagues, including everyone at GCMHP, who have supported, and worked with him over the years. I am reluctant to provide a shortlist for fear of missing people out. However, I'm sure those of you out there reading this will know your impact on Eyad's life and how grateful he was. Finally, the book started as a non-profit venture, and no proceeds from sales of this book will go to me/the author. Instead, proceeds will support both the publisher, Daraja Press, whose goals I believe align with Eyad's core values and GCMHP.

It's a great pain that Eyad was unable to read this work; I can't sit down over coffee to discuss it with him. However, at his favourite café in Gaza, I can imagine both of us leafing through printed pages of the book as we decided what to keep and what to add. It's hard to know what he would think of the outcome, but I hope he would have given his typical and encouraging smile of approval.

PROLOGUE

In 2008, in response to Operation Cast Lead (Israel's war on Gaza), like any young Western activist, I started a Facebook group. The Facebook group had no real aim and would soon become one of many derelict online spaces. But I found myself enthused to be jostling with others online. I was getting 'likes' for speaking up for what felt right. At the time, I was working as a recruitment consultant in London. It's a fast-paced sales job suited to graduates with no clearly outlined career trajectory.

I checked my Facebook group on my coffee breaks, liked other posts, and read *The Sane Society* by the humanist writer Erich Fromm. Fromm, a psychotherapist and philosopher, wrote prolifically about how capitalism and individualism can operate insidiously against our collective humanity. There was more to life, I thought, but what? In practical terms, I was worried about my dad, and existentially I was lost; going to Gaza was probably not the only, or best, option, but I was drawn to the idea.

I am leaving for Gaza as Operation Cast Lead, as Israel named it, has ended. This war on Gaza, December 2008–January 2009, was the most brutal episode of violence inflicted on Palestinians that I had witnessed and the worst since 1967. It dominated news coverage and social media, and it seemed never to end. It lasted 22 days and ultimately killed over 1400 people, of whom 400 were children.[1] It was a shocking act of violence. The stated aim was to combat rocket fire from Gaza into Israel. Given the asymmetry of warfare and near-total control Israel has on Gaza, it's hard to believe that Israel could eliminate rocket fire by indiscriminately dropping bombs on swathes of Gaza. The policy was callously referred to as 'mowing the grass.'[2] Indeed, the aim was to sow fear into Gazans and remind Hamas, the newly elected political party, that they were not, and would never be, in control? This war was a harbinger of the future.

Not long later, I very aimlessly left London. However, the one thing I recall doing was buying some sort of hiking shoes, anticipating that I would be walking over rubble and sand. In hindsight, it was a purchase that revealed how dislocated from life in Gaza I was. I would later learn that the more common shoe – at least among my class – in Gaza was more of a smart suede loafer. This dress attire also spoke to an Arab gentry. One that is often entirely overlooked by Western media, who prefer to imagine only sandal-wearing Palestinians. I left for Heathrow airport, with my comfortable hiking shoes and some books by the political writer Noam Chomsky.

Travelling in and out of Palestine is not as simple as booking a flight. Of course, I have a British passport, but I was also born in Gaza. On a trip to Gaza in 2006, Israeli officials only granted me entry on the condition that I obtained an *Hawiyya* (a Palestinian ID Card issued by Israel). That summer, I was visiting my family and faced an unjust dilemma. Either I accepted their conditions, or I couldn't enter Palestine. I was left with no choice and took up this green ID card. This card renders me a Palestinian, and for Israel at least, trumps my British citizenship. With my new *Hawiyya*, I am a *real* Palestinian and at the mercy of Israel's mood and security apparatus.

Concerning my movement, there isn't a clear set of defined rules or an online platform that reveals a comforting green tick to demonstrate you are permitted entry. Getting in and out of Palestine is a black box. Inside the black box are a network of relations, whose actors often communicate by SMS to deny or accept your entry. Of course, it helps to know people; the Arabic for this nepotism or having connections is *wasta*. My father being who he is, meant I had some *wasta*. Still, I am leaving for Palestine in the knowledge that Israel – like for all travellers to Israel – is entirely in control of my movements in and out of Palestine.

For Israel, due to my ancestry, I am not British. They try to tease out my lineage at the border: Who is your father? Who is your grandfather? Some of the younger Israeli soldiers are confused by my polished English accent and chinos: 'Are you a diplomat?' one asked. When I describe how my Palestinian DNA impacts my movements in Palestine, people are surprised. Many British people assume that being British is a universal trump card. Perhaps it's due to Britain's previous role as the global superpower, a cultural legacy that makes many British feel so powerful and central to everything.

A further twist to the story of Israel's control of my movements is that I was born in Israel. My mother went into premature labour and gave birth in a hospital in Ashkelon. On the official birth certificate, it says, in Hebrew, something to the effect that I was born *in transit*. This linguistic trick is a way to prevent me from taking up rights to any Israeli citizenship. All official government IDs, including my British passport, wrongly state that I was born in Gaza. The complete control of my movement is a feature of Israel's occupation. It is a significant theme of the lives of Palestinians, one that has only worsened over the years.

Arrival

It's March 2009, Obama is now in office, and I arrive at Cairo airport. As I passed through airport security, almost comically lax, I placed a Noam Chomsky book: 'The Fateful Triangle' on the conveyor belt. The book is about US-Palestine-Israel relations. An older white American man, wearing a Panama hat, saw the book, looked up, and said: 'You should be careful with that sort of book here.' I replied jovially that he should read it. To which he said mysteriously: 'In another life, perhaps.' Maybe he was in the CIA, I pondered.

Of course, American power over the region was omnipresent. Later that year, in June, Obama gave a speech in Cairo. He carefully laid out his vision for the Middle East in the address. He was trying to signal to the world that he was not George Bush Jr and wanted the world to know he wasn't interested in starting more wars. He also had words of encouragement for Palestinians and sterner words for Israel.[3] His speech set a more hopeful tone and signalled that things would be different this time.

In Zamalek, an aristocratic neighbourhood in Cairo where my relatives live, I am waiting for an email from Eyad. I am waiting for news telling me if I am on 'the list'. The list is a daily list of people allowed into Palestine via the Rafah border. Eyad, via his contacts in the Egyptian military, eventually tells me I have been granted permission: I can leave for Gaza tomorrow. There is only one way to get to Rafah, via car or bus. So, I undertake a four-to-five-hour car trip across the Sinai. My driver is an Egyptian who has attached a digital TV monitor to his dashboard to keep himself entertained. His favourite shows, he tells me, are history. I spend the next four hours declining Marlboro Red cigarettes, dodging oncoming cars, and watching a History Channel documentary on the 1967 Arab war.

We arrived at the Rafah border. Rafah is the Egyptian-controlled entry to Palestine, but over which Israel has official oversight. My entry was 'coordinated' by my father. The absence of any formal application system is anxiety-provoking. You arrive at these big gates, which in Europe are now historical tourist attractions, not literal gateways for people, without any paperwork. I am just hoping my name, as was promised, is on 'the list'. You wait with other crowds of Palestinians. There are local Egyptian children, often shoeless and begging. As one person commented to me before leaving: you will now see how two-thirds of the world live. At Rafah, both Palestinians' and Egyptians' poverty and utter desperation are raw. There is tension and a sense of resignation in the air.

Once inside the gates, you pass through what is essentially passport control. It's tense, you don't know what is happening, and to make matters worse, you can see Palestine. You can quite literally see the grass blades of the other side, like a prisoner glimpsing freedom. The irony was that I was going from one sense of oppression to another—but at least I would be home.

Time passes, and you shuffle around biding your time. The Egyptian security doesn't update you as they take their time processing your paperwork. They are probably waiting for Israel to give the green light. It's a familiar sense of anxiety and an awareness that your denial of entry will have no accountability or process of recourse. I look around at other despondent, tired Palestinians. Some look incredibly smart in shirts and ties, others in Western-looking sweatpants, and many in comfortable clothes. Ones that to Westerners would probably resemble the stereotypical garments of the 'poor'. As I look around the room, I wonder where they have been and what they are going back to? If they are out of Gaza, why go back?

I reach a part of the terminal where you have to pay for your three-minute bus ride to the 'Palestinian side'. The whole system is a racket. A bus, in much need of a service, is overfilled, and bags are slung onto a trolley attached to the back. The whole thing takes you a few minutes. You have no choice but to pay the fees. In my stupidity, I had run out of cash in the relevant currency on this occasion. I was alone in the terminal without any money. Thankfully I was around other Palestinians, so in this sense, I was not alone. This is what community can look and feel like. A middle-aged man overhears my conversation, and without hesitation, he lends me the money. It was about three or five dollars. He doesn't know me, only my family name. I would learn that this act of solidarity, generosity and graciousness is a hallmark of Palestinian culture.

I finally arrived at the Palestinian side. I feel calmer because I know I won't be turned back to Egypt by Palestinians. These are 'my people' but you have to go through what feels like the performative role of a very new state (Hamas) seeking to demonstrate its new power and authority. My bags are going through the typical security conveyor belt. A bearded Hamas official looks on with what appears like seriousness that serves to inflate his feeling of authority. I wondered what it's like for these men, who had been in some cases jailed, not only by Israel but also by the Palestinian Authority, to now be exerting power over other Palestinians.

My things exit the conveyor belt, and a big man with a neat beard (since Hamas, these neat beards are more prevalent in Gaza) takes me to one side. He speaks to me in Arabic; my Arabic is very poor. He is confused, and I am embarrassed. After all, I am a Sarraj (a well-known Palestinian family), but I don't speak Arabic. Over the years, I have learned that being Palestinian and not speaking Arabic is considered a matter of shame. I have stopped counting the number of people from all over the Arab world who voluntarily show their disappointment learning I don't speak Arabic.

The guard is in front of me, leafing through my Chomsky books but obviously not reading them. He then asks me where my mum and dad are from. I say my dad is from Gaza, and my mum is English. He seems confused but then brazenly asks me their religion. I tell him my dad is Muslim and my mum is Christian. Confused, his logic forces him to ask me which religion is better. I pause and reply: Islam? He agrees with a shake of his head, and I nervously mutter – as if my loyalty is in question – something like *'beheb* Gaza' (I love Gaza). Hamas is in charge, and they are making things unnecessarily tense.

I am in Gaza now: it's a massive relief from the stress of the day's constant anxiety and uncertainty. I am met by Samir, my dad's loyal and trusted friend. Samir is a refugee. He lives in a refugee camp and has seven kids. As well as being a father, he is a talented drummer. He is a genius with engineering, funny, kind and highly resourceful. He often asked me to get him electrical items from abroad, but not ones 'made in China' – he thinks they don't last as long.

He was a dear friend to my dad and an incredibly decent and honest man. What I always admired was his remarkable ability to be cheerful and playful. But he is human, and, I noticed with sadness, this quality faded, as life under siege in Gaza took its toll. We drive along the coast towards Remal (the area where my father lives).

We arrive at the house, and I open the large iron door. My dad walks toward me. His walk is not bountiful, and he is slower. It's cold in Gaza today. He is wearing a shell suit and baseball cap. He could be both fashionable and completely nonchalant about clothing, preferring to wear whatever makes him feel comfortable. He is wearing the very same outfit I had seen him wear the day before on the BBC. He gives me a tight hug, and we go into the house.

Eyad had been all over TV in the weeks before. He was advocating to 'end the siege',[4] an attempt to raise awareness of the effects of the crippling siege. Ending the siege had galvanized him again. He loved Gaza, loved Palestine, and that's what he did. He was committed to improving life in Gaza. He would take up any interview, media appearance, or writing obligation, but never with any view to promoting anything other than the improvement of Palestine. He wasn't carefully crafting a persona, or media image. It was raw, from the heart. He rarely, if ever, spoke from notes. It was mostly all from lived experience and a clear sense of justice.

When he learned how I was treated at the border, he said: 'thick head...I will call his boss'. This was Eyad. He had power and connections. He would get a phone call, a meeting over tea, with this officer's boss. The conversation would be logical: why is your employee doing this? Many of those high up in Hamas were intelligent and thoughtful. In 2009, they wanted to be part of the 'international community'. Unfortunately, some of those lower down in Hamas did what they might think their bosses would like. Eyad knew how Hamas treating people like this at the borders would damage international relations and sow unhelpful seeds. Eyad knew how important foreigners visiting Gaza were. I also mentioned how I had been lent a few dollars at the border. Eyad looked at Samir, spoke in Arabic, and, with very little information to go on, knew how to find him.

I hadn't long been in Gaza, but you soon realize how complicated and interconnected things are: Egypt's role in securing my entry, the scale of poverty, the destruction caused by Operation Cast Lead, the kinship between Palestinians and the new role that Hamas would be taking on under Obama's careful watch and the grassroots campaign to end the siege on Gaza. Amidst all this was Eyad. He was now 66, had remarried and had a new young son aged five, and was receiving treatment for Multiple Myeloma (a blood cancer). Who was my father? How did he become the first psychiatrist in the Gaza Strip? Why was this calm, reasonable man imprisoned and tortured by Arafat? How did he go from medical student to an international writer, speaker, advocate, activist, and whose obituary appeared in the *New York Times*?[5]

Eyad Rajab Sarraj was not born until 1944, four years before the creation of Israel. So, to better understand him and the world he was entering, it's necessary to go back to the late 19th Century.

Notes

1. Amnesty International 2009, 'Israel/Gaza: Operation "Cast Lead": 22 days of death and destruction', <https://www.amnesty.org/en/documents/mde15/015/2009/en/>
2. Rabbani, M 2014, 'Israel Mows the Lawn', *London Review of Books*, July 31st, <https://www.lrb.co.uk/the-paper/v36/n15/mouin-rabbani/israel-mows-the-lawn>
3. Obama, B 2009. *The President's Speech in Cairo: A New Beginning*, Cairo University, Cairo, June 4th
4. 'Free Gaza Founder Eyad Sarraj responds to Netanyahu and Barak 2010', 2010, online video, viewed October 1st, 2021 <https://www.youtube.com/watch?v=ceIggX9LZDg>
5. Akram, F 2013, 'Eyad El-Sarraj, Psychiatrist Who Fought for Palestinians' Rights, Dies at 70', New York Times, December 18th <https://www.nytimes.com/2013/12/19/world/middleeast/eyad-el-sarraj-psychiatrist-who-fought-for-rights-of-palestinians-is-dead-at-70.html>

1. EMPIRES AND TRIBES

It's easy to overlook that states are human creations. It can be hard to imagine the world as not always being 195 countries that regularly compete in things like the World Cup or the Olympic Games. However, before nation-states, there were things like empires and caliphates. These were different ways of holding vast swathes of land, collecting taxes, and using force to control large populations. Palestine and Israel, as states, are 20th Century creations.

Historically, the area known as Palestine (the area between the Mediterranean Sea and the Jordan River) was at a crossroads between three continents. It was subject to multiple invasions and, over time, had many different rulers. In the most recent times, before Israel and Palestine existed as nation-states, the area's rulers were the British and the Ottoman Empire before them. Palestine being at this geographical crossroads led to layer upon layer of human interactions. Over time this dynamic led to the development of a rich culture. Pamela Ann Smith, the historian, describes Palestine in the 19th Century:

> ... the patchwork quilt of different cultures, religions and ways of life, spawned by the endless waves of invasion, had produced a network of anarchic bonhomie where Maghiribi mystics, Armenian craftsmen, Talmudic scholars, British mercenaries, Turkish gendarmerie and Greek orthodox traders lived side by side with the merchants, landowners and religious elite.[1]

Palestine, before 1917, sounds like a modern city. In today's terms, we might call it a melting pot to appreciate its diversity. But it also serves as an important reminder of how Palestine *was* diverse. It speaks to a tolerance of others that we often sadly don't associate with Palestine, or perhaps even more tragically with humanity itself. However, this tolerance and diversity come as no surprise to me. Without exception I, and non-Palestinian, even Jewish, friends, have been treated with such generosity by Palestinians. I recall being invited to the home of Palestinian refugees in Gaza. Despite the extremely limited resources and cramped living conditions, they went out of their way to make us fresh banana and strawberry smoothies. A treat for them and a gift for us. This is very much the norm, and many visitors to Palestine will have similar stories of such gracious acts of hospitality.

The Ottoman Empire was the most recent empire to preside over the geographical area known as Palestine. Between the 14th and early 20th Century, the

Ottoman Empire was a Turkish empire that, at its peak, controlled much of Southeastern Europe, Western Asia, and Northern Africa. Its control of Palestine was to last – almost uninterrupted – from 1516 until the early 20th Century.

However, although the Ottoman Empire ruled Palestine, exactly how power was administered locally was far more complex. It wasn't simply top-down instructions from the head of the Ottoman Empire. It was more like Historic Palestine was a collection of families, clans, and tribes. While in competition with each other, these clans also had sophisticated mechanisms of arbitration and reconciliation that allowed peace to be a mainstay of the region. Indeed, my father and his Israeli friend tried to use these exact mechanisms (*a hudna*) to reconcile Hamas, Fatah and Israel.[2]

These clans amassed power and established ownership of things like soap factories, vegetable gardens, bakeries etc. All the things you would need to survive, make money and build authority. Their power was so great that, in some cases, the clans were even able to appoint members of their clan to the position of Ottoman governor. This mutually beneficial relationship between the clans and the Ottomans allowed taxes to keep rolling in and peace to be maintained.

This system of clan power did not last forever. A significant turning point in Palestinian history was the shift from families sharing in the cultivation of land (that is to say, the profits from things they grew) to one where families owned the land and employed people to cultivate the land. This meant that those who owned the land made the money, and those who tilled it made much less. The consequence of this new system was that families – and not the wider clan – started to amass land and power. For example, the Barghoutis owned 39 villages. The Shawa family of Gaza had 100,000 dunums. A Jewish family, the Bergheims, owned 20,000.[3] This was to foreshadow a future in which family tribes would grow in dominance.

This clan history may sound fantastical, like the TV show Game of Thrones, but its relevance to modern Palestine remains central. When you live in a place like Gaza, family surnames take on far greater importance. When I lived in Gaza, I knew members of the Shawa family. I had taught their children at the American School in Gaza, a private fee-paying school for the well-off to send their children. I had also known the Shawa family as butchers. I would order BBQ kebab with herbs and spices, warm pita bread, grilled tomatoes, and onion from their restaurant. It was one of my, and my father's, favourite things to eat in Gaza. Eyad often observed the contradictory role the tribal structure in Palestine played. While he followed them, they offered protection, conflict resolution (*Solha*), and security. He also lamented their role in undermining the state's ability to provide law and order. That is to say, the state did not have a monopoly on power.

Politics of Notables

Power in Palestine in the 19th Century was primarily dispersed through clans and families who had, in some part, good relationships with the ruling Ottoman empire. These families are commonly known as 'notable families', and they developed power through their relationships with the *ashraf* ('men of the pen'). The *ashraf* were men who claimed to be descendants of the Prophet Muhammad or of great military commanders who had led early Islamic conquests in the 7th Century.[4] Their power and wealth came from their control of the *awqaf* (charitable estates). Over time the *ashraf* formed alliances with 'notable families' such as the Hussainis, Khalidis, Nashashibis and Jarallahs. The two groups became virtually indistinguishable. The alliance led to members of these families being given access to state positions in the civil service, army and educational institutions. The children of these families benefited from modern education and learning new languages.[5]

The Sarraj family was not powerful in the same way as the previously mentioned families. However, they did occupy positions of authority. My great grandfather was a well-respected religious figure. My great uncle Jameel El Sarraj was the Chief Justice of Jaffa. And the Sarraj family also included a Chief of Police. My grandfather, Rajab Sarraj, was born in Beersheba and would go on to work in the British Police Force. All these roles meant the Sarraj family had security through income and relationships. However, they did not own vast swathes of land, nor did they own factories. They were a small and intellectual family.

The other important facet of the Sarraj family is that they were from Gaza. In historic Islamic literature, Gaza was known as 'Ghazzat Hashem', Hashem's Gaza. Hashem ibn 'Abd Manaf is the grandfather of the Prophet Muhammad and is buried in 'Sayed al-Hashim Mosque' in ad-Darraj Quarter of the Old City in Gaza.[6] This alone marks Gaza as an incredibly important religious site. Of course, Palestinians do identify as one people. Still, many Palestinians have continuously resided in Gaza and were later joined by refugees fleeing from other parts of Palestine. This led to the refugee/non-refugee divide in Gaza. Gaza today is host to 2.1 million people, 1.4 million of whom are refugees.

Tracing the origins of the Sarrajs beyond Gaza and the Ottomans is no small task. But clues perhaps lie with my father's fondness for Granada, Spain. When we visited the famous Alhambra palace (*The Red One*), a mid-13th Century Royal Palace for Yusuf, the Sultan of Granada – instead of ignoring the customary tourist photos, and to all our surprise – he gleefully leapt at the opportunity. I never imagined seeing him reclining on a chaise longue, looking delighted and wearing the full regalia of that period, complete with a bejewelled curved sword known as a scimitar. At that time, I was a mortified teenager, and my dad was dressed up like he was an extra in Disney's Aladdin. But, looking back, it serves as a friendly reminder of his playful side and would also have been a moment for him to be away from the stress and strain of Gaza.

His connection to Granada, and his values, may well have been in his DNA. I discovered that the Abencerrages, the Arabic for Saddler's Son, were a Moor family who, during the 15th Century, held prominent positions in the Kingdom of Granada. The family is known for its 'elegance, good grace, disposition and bravery'.[7] One story told from this period is about Abindarráez, a young scion of the Abencerrajes, who falls in love with Jarifa. It's a story about a Christian and a Muslim who work together as they strive to see virtue and honour in each other. It's a tale of tolerance, friendship and understanding across religious lines.

Notes

1. Smith, P 1984, *Palestine and the Palestinians - 1876-1983*, St Martin's Press, New York, pp8
2. Erlich, E 2018, 'Only a Reconciliation Delegation Will Bring About a Cease-fire', *Haaretz*, June 19th
3. Smith, P 1984, *Palestine and the Palestinians - 1876-1983*, St Martin's Press, New York, pp13
4. ibid
5. Khalidi, R 2020, *The Hundred Years' War on Palestine: A History of Settler Colonialism and Resistance, 1917–2017*, Metropolitan Books, New York, pp18
6. Filiu, J 2014, *Gaza: A History*, Hurst & Company, London, pp32
7. Fuchs, B 2014, *The Abencerraje and Ozmin and Daraja,* University of Pennsylvania Press, US, pp32

2. THE BRITISH

Throughout the 19th Century, the British were engaged in a 'Peaceful Crusade' of the Middle East.[1] For example, the British Consulate was built in Jerusalem in 1838, a form of 'soft power'. As methods and cost of travel developed, there was an increase in travel from Britain to Palestine. As a result, the view of Palestine in Britain was evolving from an almost mythical place to physical reality – a place you could go.

Despite British interest in Palestine, the Ottomans were still controlling the region. However, World War I had precipitated war between the Ottomans and the British. The British, or *Ingliz*, as they were known in Arabic, were now at war with the Ottomans, who had recruited Palestinians on horseback to defend against the invading *Ingliz*. As a result, there were three infamous battles of Gaza, the first two resulting in losses for the British. To change tack, the British appointed a new commander General Allenby. He successfully led the British to victory in the third battle by launching a surprise attack on Beersheba.

Being half British, I read this history with mixed feelings. Gaza and Beersheba are names that are known to me as my father's home and his place of birth, respectively. They are not in my mind 'places of battle' or ones that stoke feelings of 'victory'. On the contrary, these wars would have spread fear amongst my ancestors and left them with life-or-death choices. Tragically, current generations face the same decision whether to stay, fight or flee Gaza. In this sense, '*Ingliz*' to my family in Palestine is not a word that necessarily fills them with joy. On the contrary, they blame what has happened to Palestine on the '*Ingliz*'.

The British casualties from these wars are still commemorated in Gaza itself. I visited the British Cemetery in the South, a Commonwealth Grave host to 3,217 burials from the First and Second World Wars.[2] On visiting, what surprised me was how well it was looked after. Lush, deep green grass and almost perfectly aligned gravestones. It's perhaps a minor point but a reminder that despite the overwhelmingly negative stories of Gaza in the media, there is a groundsman who tends carefully to these lawns and a local community who respects the cemetery's existence. Gaza is not full of 'barbarians'.[3]

Balfour and Zionism

As the British, and the French, grew confident that they would defeat the Ottomans, they agreed to a 'secret treaty' known as Sykes-Picot. This agreement was signed in 1916 that meant after the Ottomans were defeated, they would divide up the former Ottoman provinces along British and French lines. In addition to other areas, the UK were to be allocated what we know today as Israel, Palestine, and Jordan.

Sure enough, on October 31st, 1917, Beersheba, where Eyad was born and situated outside the Gaza region, fell to the British. Two days after this, the British Foreign Secretary, Arthur James Balfour, issued a letter known as the Balfour Declaration. By December 1917, Jerusalem was occupied, marking 1,300 years of Islamic rule in Palestine. The Prime Minister of Britain at that time was Lloyd George, who in 1931 spoke about the meaning of the Balfour declaration:

> By the terms of that document recognition was given to the historical connection of the Jewish people with Palestine, and the grounds for reconstituting their National Home in that country.[4]

Jewish migration to Palestine had been happening for many years during the Ottoman period. Antisemitic pogroms in the Russian Empire left Jewish populations with no choice but to flee. Approximately 15,000 Jewish settlers came to Palestine from the early 1880s until 1904, and 30,000 by 1914. Between 1880–1914 30 Zionist colonies were established in Palestine. Zionism's central pillar was that Judaism was both a nationality and a religion. Jews would have the right to their own homeland/nation-state. This idea of a home for Jews was taking shape when states, or independent nations, became a feature of the world order and amidst rising antisemitism.[5]

Antisemitism was a scourge on Europe and took different forms. It included things like Jews not being able to get specific jobs. Jews were fighting not only violent persecution but also structural racism. Many Jews were left-wing, and they wanted to overthrow the existing system for a fairer one. The history of leftist thought and fighting this kind of oppression in Europe can sometimes be overlooked. I would later become friends with and meet many Jews in Palestine and the UK, pro-Palestinian, anti-Zionist and left-wing.

Palestine was not always the destination for a Jewish homeland. Theodor Herzl, one of the founders of Zionism, had even considered Argentina. Learning that the 'founders of Zionism' were considering Argentina as a home for Jews serves as a reminder that nothing was written in stone. Instead, people had to make decisions and think through options. Deciding on Palestine was a decision.

However, it was only with the resources and power of the British that a home for Jews could have come to fruition.

The Zionist movement, led by Theodor Herzl, had finally acquired the help of a great power. The British had decided to use their power to help the Jewish people establish a 'home' in Palestine. 'Palestine' or 'Arab' is not even mentioned in the entire Balfour document. It's also clear that a very negative view of Palestine had formed in the minds of The British establishment.[6] They thought that Palestinians were not economically prosperous and that their land was simply filled with malaria.[7] They, of course, used these views as one of their justifications for creating a home for the Jewish people. However, recent scholarship has demonstrated to the contrary that Palestine at this time was undergoing rapid transitions.[8]

The term that is often used to describe what was happening is: 'settler colonialism'. It's an academic term that means that local inhabitants, in this case, Palestinians, are forcibly removed or killed, i.e., with violence, to 'settle' a new people. As Rashid Khalidi clarifies, Britain, for its geopolitical interests, found that its goals overlapped with the Zionists: it was a mutually beneficial relationship, one not based on altruism.[9]

Sir Herbert Samuel, a prominent British Zionist, was appointed to High Commissioner of the Palestine Mandate.[10] By now, the British had lent their support to both Zionism and Arab independence. It's a sort of hubris, brazenness, and dishonesty that perhaps best characterizes the UK's current Prime Minister Boris Johnson.[11] This is not a cheap point: the nature of acting without due care seems endemic in certain parts of UK political culture. Nevertheless, the ensuing chaos from these contradictory promises led to Winston Churchill, the Colonial Secretary, visiting Palestine and Gaza in 1921, and in a speech often quoted, he said:

> It is manifestly right that the Jews, who are scattered all over the world, should have a national center and a national home where some of them may be reunited. And where else could that be but in this land of Palestine, with which for more than 3,000 years they have been intimately and profoundly associated? We think it will be good for the world, good for the Jews and good for the British Empire. But we also think it will be good for the Arabs who dwell in Palestine.[12]

Crowds had gathered in Gaza to witness Churchill's arrival, and he was greeted by waving Palestinians. But this was not jubilation: the reality was that Palestinians saw him as an envoy for the Balfour declaration. A declaration that had given up Palestine to other people and laid the ground for a hundred-year war. As Edward Said put it in his book *The Question of Palestine*:

> ...a plain and irreducible core of the Palestinian experience for the last hundred years [is] that on the land called Palestine there existed as a huge

majority for hundreds of years a largely pastoral, a nevertheless socially, culturally, politically, economically identifiable people whose language and religion were (for a huge majority) Arabic and Islam, respectively. This people—or, if one wishes to deny them any modern conception of themselves as a people, this group of people—identified itself with the land it tilled and lived on (poorly or not is irrelevant), the more so after an almost wholly European decision was made to resettle, reconstitute, recapture the land for Jews who were to be brought there from elsewhere... such as it is, the Palestinian actuality is today, was yesterday, and most likely tomorrow will be built upon an act of resistance to this new foreign colonialism.[13]

Life Under the British

Rajab Sarraj, my grandfather, was originally from Gaza—although the Sarraj family itself moved around Palestine, settling in cities (which are all today in Israel) such as Jaffa, Haifa and Acre. These urban centres were proliferating, and by the end of the British Mandate period, both Jaffa and Haifa had a larger Arab population than Jerusalem.

My earliest memory of my grandfather was seeing him in his garden in Gaza. He was skinny but healthy and tanned. He was wearing a light pink jallabiya. He always seemed very gentle, kind and softly spoken. I recall my mother, who is English, remembering specifically how kind, honourable and decent he was. She had struggled with the cultural differences in Gaza, and my grandfather was a source of support throughout her time in Gaza.

My grandfather was educated in Jaffa and, at 20 years old, managed to find work in Beersheba. However, he was only here briefly before marrying and starting a family in Jaffa. He had never met his future wife, but according to my father, he fell in love at first sight. My grandfather eventually moved back to Beersheba in 1939 to take up a new job. Beersheba at that time was lush. According to the British explorer Edward Hull, its abundance of crops and natural beauty reminded him of Southern Italy. Not a comparison you often hear when thinking of Palestine, but a reminder of Palestine's undeniable beauty.

My grandfather continued to work diligently and ended up on a good salary working as the Chief Clerk for the British Mandate Police Force. He dreamed of settling in Gaza. To achieve this goal, he regularly sent money to his father-in-law, who had been instructed to build a family home in Remal. My grandfather's job in the British Police was a source of security that allowed him to prepare for this future. In oral testimony, a Palestinian villager recalls:

...one of the jobs available to villagers was to be employed by the government in the police. Many villagers took up this work, some reaching quite high positions. It was like a hereditary job — when the father was a policeman the sons would follow him.[14]

With Rajab in gainful work, he was able to establish some security. The Sarraj family were relatively small and was not a large clan. The British (like the Ottomans) were aware of powerful clans and families and sought to control society through them. They dished out positions to wealthy and land-owning families and used divide-and-rule tactics. They also sought to play families off one another. In Gaza, the British were able to control the local families and sowed division between families like the Souranis and Shawas. At one point Said Shawa, Deputy Mayor of Gaza was even imprisoned by the British.[15]

While Rajab dreamed of returning to Gaza, Gaza struggled to rebuild itself after Allenby's troops had triumphantly marched through. This tragic thread of Gaza having to rebuild itself and manage infighting, sowed and fueled, by powerful occupiers is profoundly depressing and revealing. Power has been utilized throughout the generations to undermine efforts by Palestinians to become more united, organized, and powerful.

Police Brutality

The British Mandate Police Force, where my grandfather worked, was a brutal colonial force. It was a force that attracted former soldiers, initially from the British paramilitary 'Black and Tans' who were deployed against Irish rebels in the early 1920s. This 'paramilitary' style force also reportedly attracted men who were on the 'margins of society'. These types of men were recruited as it was thought that they would act outside of any law and would perhaps relish the opportunity to administer violence.[16]

They reportedly hated the population they were policing and drank heavily. It was often said that the police were more brutal than the army. The British adopted the 'Turkish Method' of policing, which meant they outsourced policing to local Arabs, Jews and other non-British groups. This outsourcing led to Arabs inflicting violence on other Arabs.

When a British police officer witnessed Arab police beating three suspects and applying lit cigarettes to their testicles, he later asked the British commanding officer what was going on:

> ... force was the only language these Arabs understood. Under Turkish rule they had been brought up to respect such methods. 'Where do you think we would get,' he asked me 'if we questioned them like a London bobby?

I'll tell you; the police methods would be laughed at, we should get no results, and our methods would be regarded as a sign of weakness.' 'In these interrogations,' he went on, 'I make it a rule never to beat anyone up myself. I let Arab police beat up Arabs, and Jewish police beat up Jews.[17]

Douglas Duff, a policeman, went on to describe how the police would deal with a Palestinian crowd disturbance:

Had our Arabic been better we might have sympathized with them; though I doubt it, for most of us were so infected by the sense of our own superiority over 'lesser breeds' that we scarcely regarded these people as human...Police officers in vehicles would try to knock down Arabs, 'as running over an Arab is the same as a dog in England except we do not report it.[18]

Discussions of colonialism, for many, may conjure up visions of slavery. However, this can obscure the precise nature of colonial occupation in Palestine. The British had a brutal system of control set up in Palestine, which they had already tested in other countries. What is evident from the British practices is that they were to be the start of a thread of violence and dehumanization inflicted on Palestinians.

There are clear parallels in how the British police described Arabs and how many Israeli officers talk about Palestinians. Overall, it's a language that justifies the most vicious acts on largely defenceless people. Eyad would spend much of his professional life trying to understand the implications of violence and dehumanization. And in a modest way, try to heal these wounds at both the individual and community level.

Amidst British control, life continued: Gaza continued to grow and was a bustling place filled with bazaars. Its population in the late 1920s was 17,000, today it is 2.1 million.[19] Gaza was also benefitting from the actions of its mayor: Fahmi al-Husseini. He had embarked on a series of urban improvements which led to the development of a bright modern suburb: Remal (the sands). This would be where my father and his father would eventually settle. Remal was always considered a safe and affluent area. Eyad tried to beautify his community. In the 1990s, Eyad was so keen on this that he managed to get the local municipality to plant trees along his road, ones that still exist today.

Revolution

In 1922 the League of Nations, the precursor to the United Nations, had formalized Britain's control of Palestine. The League of Nations upheld the commitments laid out in the Balfour Declaration. But, according to Palestinian historian

Rashid Khalidi, the League of Nations implied that the only people in Palestine to be recognized with national rights were the Jewish people. It is also clear that the document sought to describe Jewish people as the only people to have a historical connection to Palestine. This, in effect, erased thousands of years of history dating past the Ottoman Empire. And as Khalidi notes: 'the surest way to eradicate a people's right to their land is to deny their historical connection to it.'[20] The stage was set for war.

By 1935, things were reaching a tipping point in Palestine. The Jewish population in Palestine had risen from 61,000 in 1919 to 355,000 by 1935. The Jewish population now represented nearly 30% of the total population.[21] And elite led initiatives by notable Palestinians to reconcile with the Jewish community in Palestine had been fruitless. In this context, Sheikh Izzeldin al Qassam, a Muslim preacher based in Haifa, led a small armed militia known as the Black Hand Group. He declared a rebellion against British rule and went to battle with them.

British troops killed him, and his death sparked an outcry in the villages and towns. This man killed in 1935 was to have a long legacy. It's his name that Hamas' military wing takes as their own: the Qassam Brigades. Of course, the shifting contexts make it hard to draw direct comparisons between Hamas today and what Qassam's goals and strategy were. However, that his name carries on demonstrates the deep roots of political violence in Palestine and the ongoing nature of resistance to occupation.

In April 1936, armed followers of Qassam killed two Jews near Tulkarem. This led to a militant Jewish group killing two Arab workers near Jaffa. More violence broke out, followed by a general Arab workers' strike across Palestine. As an act of solidarity and commitment to a unified goal, the Palestinian political parties formed a joint leadership known as the Arab Higher Committee (AHC). The AHC was led by the Mufti of Jerusalem and united notable Palestinian families. These events culminated in what is known as the 'Arab Revolt', or in Arabic *thawra* (revolution). The death toll of this revolution by mid-October of 1936 was 1,000 Palestinians, 80 Jews, and 37 British.[22]

It was a confluence of factors that was now about to shift the political realities more extreme. World War II had started, and the British, post Arab Revolt, realized that they would not be able to maintain a significant force in Palestine to control the Arab population. So in 1939, the British issued something called a 'White Paper', which is essentially a document that makes a series of recommendations to a government. This 1939 White Paper stated:

> His Majesty's Government believe that the framers of the Mandate in which the Balfour Declaration was embodied could not have intended that Palestine should be converted into a Jewish State against the will of the Arab population of the country....His Majesty's Government therefore now declare unequivocally that it is not part of their policy that Pales-

tine should become a Jewish State. They would indeed regard it as contrary to their obligations to the Arabs under the Mandate, as well as to the assurances which have been given to the Arab people in the past, that the Arab population of Palestine should be made the subjects of a Jewish State against their will.

The objective of His Majesty's Government is the establishment within 10 years of an independent Palestine State in such treaty relations with the United Kingdom as will provide satisfactorily for the commercial and strategic requirements of both countries in the future...The independent State should be one in which Arabs and Jews share government in such a way as to ensure that the essential interests of each community are safeguarded.[23]

Palestinians rejected the paper's recommendations, and Britain's promises were met with understandable scepticism. But what the paper had done was rile Zionists. It had, very importantly, stated that Jewish immigration to Palestine would be limited to 75,000. This was a trigger for far greater Zionist organized violence against the British. This violence was carried out by Zionist paramilitary groups such as the Irgun and Hagganah. However, as World War II took shape and fighting took hold of North Africa, Britain worried it would lose ground to the Germans. So in a tactical move, it armed Zionists and made sure arms flowed to their military groups.

With more arms flowing to Zionists, a new Jewish group emerged called the LEHI 'Fighters for The Freedom of Israel'. This group was more radical, considered Britain more of an enemy than the Arabs and called for an end to the Mandate. This splintering of political groups within Zionism reflected both the complexity and uncertainty of the moment. Britain wanted Zionism as a source of regional stability but faced violent attacks. It was, in many ways, struggling to have everything going its way on its terms. World War II was about to usher in a new world order, and Britain would no longer enjoy its control of the world.

Generational Trauma

The violence that Zionists were carrying out against the British cannot be looked at in isolation. During 1941-44, 6 million Jews were killed in the Holocaust. In this context, fear of British defeat, and the possibility of Germans taking Palestine, were real. In the event of Nazis arriving in Palestine, young Jews were reported to be considering mass suicide. Another significant event was the sinking of the Struma. This was a boat that set sail from Romania with nearly 800 Jews on board. It aimed to reach the safety of Palestine. The ship reached Turkey; engine failure, and the refusal of the British to let the boat land in Palestine, meant that the vessel was towed out to sea and left floating in the Mediterranean. The boat, lost at sea, with no engine, filled with desperate families, was then torpedoed by a Soviet submarine. Only one person survived.[24]

The tragic loss of life through the Struma, and the fear gripping the Jewish community during the German invasion paint a terrifying context. It is entirely understandable that this community would be desperate for a secure and safe home. The trauma this generation has been exposed to is unimaginable. When I visit Palestine and pass Israeli checkpoints, I have to engage with the Israel Defence Forces (IDF) soldiers. These young men and women are fourth – or fifth–generation survivors of these traumas. The stories being passed down in both the Palestinian and Jewish communities are stories filled with generations of violence and dehumanization.

How these historical traumas are dealt with and processed is complicated and contested. What is clear is that there was uncertainty, paranoia, and fear during this time. In 1940, Yosef Weitz of the Jewish National Fund confided to his diary:

> ...there is no room for both people together in this country. The only solution is a Palestine ... without Arabs. And there is no other way than to transfer the Arabs from here to the neighbouring countries, to transfer all of them. There is no other way.'[25]

With Britain on the decline, Zionist leaders knew they needed more friends. World War II shifted the global balance of power, favouring the United States of America. In the early 1940s, the US began establishing military bases in the Middle East. With this knowledge, the Zionist leader, Ben Gurion, started to court US politicians and US public opinion. New York was home to a growing – and eventually, the most significant – Jewish population outside Israel. In New York, in 1942, a Zionist conference was held at the Biltmore Hotel, and a public declaration was made to create a Jewish Home in all of Palestine. US President Harry Truman subsequently endorsed this project. These events marked the shift from Britain to America, becoming the overseer of events in the region. The US would become Israel's most important supporter.[26]

With the Zionists' forces becoming more powerful and their statehood, backed by the League of Nations and the US, things looked inevitable. Many historians agree that Palestinians had been severely undermined by a powerful trio of the League of Nations, the Zionist movement, and the global powers. Some have suggested that the Palestinians should have ceased to appeal to British goodwill.[27] However, they were faced with a mighty array of forces, and perhaps there were few good options. With a weakened Palestinian side and a well-resourced and capable Zionist army, it was only a matter of time before the Zionists would take the rest of Palestine by force.

Notes

1. Polley, G 2020 *Palestine is Thus Brought Home to England: The Representation of Palestine in British Travel Literature, 1840-1914*, PhD thesis, University of Exeter, Exeter, England
2. https://www.cwgc.org/visit-us/find-cemeteries-memorials/cemetery-details/71701/gaza-war-cemetery/
3. Boyden, M 2017, 'Don't behave like Barbarians', *The Times of Israel*, Nov 5th <https://blogs.timesofisrael.com/dont-behave-like-barbarians>
4. *Jewish Telegraphic Agency* 1931, 'Mr. Lloyd George Explains Jewish National Home Policy', <https://www.jta.org/1931/04/13/archive/mr-lloyd-george-explains-jewish-national-home-policy-i-was-prime-minister-when-balfour-declaration>viewed August 5th, 2020
5. Eichler, W 2016, 'Theodor Herzl and the trajectory of Zionism', *Open Democracy*, Dec 1st
6. *Hansard* 1938, 'Palestine: Volume 341: debated on Thursday 24th November 1938' <https://hansard.parliament.uk/Commons/1938-11-24/debates/4c6147e8-c920-4b90-bfd4-d59cdda468af/Palestine>
7. ibid
8. Khalidi, R 2020, *The Hundred Years' War on Palestine: A History of Settler Colonialism and Resistance, 1917–2017*, Metropolitan Books, New York, pp20
9. ibid
10. Early Mandate Period, www.paljourneys.org, viewed <https://www.paljourneys.org/en/timeline?&sideid=173>August 5th 2021
11. Blackall, M 2021, 'Boris Johnson 'a clown' with no diplomacy skills, says ex-deputy in diaries', The Guardian, April 3rd <https://www.theguardian.com/politics/2021/apr/03/boris-johnson-a-clown-with-no-diplomacy-skills-says-ex-deputy-in-diaries>
12. Glatt, B 2016, 'Today in History: Churchill visits Mandatory Palestine', *The Jerusalem Post*, March 29th<https://www.jpost.com/christian-news/today-in-history-churchill-visits-mandatory-palestine-449569>
13. Said, E 1978, 'The Idea of Palestine in the West', *MERIP Reports* No. 70 (Sep., 1978), pp. 3-11
14. Sayigh, R 1979, *Palestinians. From Peasants to Revolutionaries*, Zed Books, London, pp6
15. Filiu, J 2014, *Gaza: A History*, Hurst & Company, London, pp102
16. Kardahji, N 2007, *A Measure of Restraint: The Palestine Police and the End of the British Mandate*, MPhil Thesis, Oxford University, Oxford, England.
17. ibid
18. ibid
19. Smith, P 1984, *Palestine and the Palestinians - 1876-1983*, St Martin's Press, New York,

pp26

20. Khalidi, R 2020, *The Hundred Years' War on Palestine: A History of Settler Colonialism and Resistance, 1917–2017*, Metropolitan Books, New York, pp34
21. Smith, P 1984, *Palestine and the Palestinians - 1876-1983*, St Martin's Press, New York, pp34
22. ibid
23. British White Paper 1939, < https://avalon.law.yale.edu/20th_century/brwh1939.asp>viewed August 5th 2020
24. Black, I 2018, *Enemies and Neighbours: Arabs and Jews in Palestine and Israel, 1917-2017*, Penguin, London, pp180
25. Black, I 2018, *Enemies and Neighbours: Arabs and Jews in Palestine and Israel, 1917-2017*, Penguin, London, pp189
26. Khalidi, R 2020, *The Hundred Years' War on Palestine: A History of Settler Colonialism and Resistance, 1917–2017*, Metropolitan Books, New York, pp59
27. Khalidi, R 2020, *The Hundred Years' War on Palestine: A History of Settler Colonialism and Resistance, 1917–2017*, Metropolitan Books, New York, pp53

3. THE *NAKBA*

> *The Palestinian inner layers of psychology go around one single issue: the 1948 uprooting and the destruction of their homes. And what the Israelis are doing, by destroying all these homes every day, they are making the Palestinians relive the trauma, which is very deeply buried into our conscious and our unconscious. The home for anybody in the world is a very important base of security, and for the Palestinians who lost their homes, once and sometimes even more than once, it is the single most important issue in the making up of the structure of psychology.*
> – Eyad Sarraj

Eyad was born in 1944, or possibly, 1943; the exact date and time are not written down, which is commonplace for Palestinians of this generation.[1] He was born in Beersheba and was to become the second eldest of nine siblings. 1944 was the same year that future Israeli Prime Minister Menachem Begin, and the leader of the Irgun (a Zionist paramilitary and terrorist organization), declared war on the British. The British and their allies had defeated the Nazis, and many, but not all, Zionists were focused on creating a safe home for Jews. Any nation – including Britain – getting in their way was an enemy. The ongoing violence against the British intensified. Assassinations were being carried out against British political figures such as Lord Moyne, who was murdered by Zionist members of LEHI (a Zionist paramilitary and terrorist organization) in Cairo.

The violence carried out by Zionists against the British was beginning to get noticed in the British media. Spectacular acts of violence, such as the bombing of the King David Hotel (causing the loss of 91 lives) and the lynching of British police caught on camera, led to antisemitic protests in Liverpool. A confluence of many factors, including these lynchings, led to a Labour government deciding to end its Mandate of Palestine and pass tenure over to the League of Nations.

According to Colonel Nichol Grey, Inspector-General of the Palestine Police:

> When the underground killed our men, we could treat it as murder; but when they erected gallows and executed our men, it was as if they were saying, 'We rule here as much as you do', and that no administration can bear. Our choice was obvious. Either total suppression or get out, and we chose the second.[2]

Rajab Sarraj, working in Beersheba, was still unaware of what was to come; he thought things in Beersheba would remain peaceful, and that life would go on. Finally, however, a local British administrator commented in November 1947:

> 'Gaza has begun to grasp that Britain is about to leave the country, but Beersheba is yet to be convinced'.[3]

The British Mandate period of Palestine was ending. This period of British rule has led to many British hallmarks lingering across the Palestinian landscape, such as the Allenby Bridge. But all these British names, Allenby, Balfour, to me, as someone growing up in the UK, are the names of things like local leisure centres, running tracks or cherry-blossom-lined streets in West London. A closer reading of the history of Palestine changes the meaning of these symbols. They are now forever tied with a much more violent history, one closer to my other home. Perhaps given this history, it would be no surprise that my father could not ever feel entirely at home in England.

Eyad was four years old in 1948. The most powerful countries in the world, including Britain, the United States and the USSR, had all agreed to the partition of Palestine. The US had decided to permit more significant Jewish migration to Israel.[4] This meant that Palestine was to be split into three parts: Arab and Jewish, while Jerusalem would be under international control. This UN resolution was numbered 181. The decision was greeted with joy by the Jewish community and dismay by the Arabs. Ben Gurion gave a speech to a large, excited crowd and proudly proclaimed: *'we are a free people'*.[5]

The narrative so far suggests a sizeable Jewish population had amassed in Palestine. In reality, Arabs still owned 90% of the country's private land, and their numbers were 1.4 million out of 2 million. Given these demographic differences, the decision to give up 55% of the country to create a Jewish state was not balanced or fair. Furthermore, the UN partition plan meant that homes belonging to Palestinians were now in Zionist territory. As a result, Palestinians would have to be forcibly removed from their home. A practice that is ongoing today.

Fleeing to Gaza

Amidst the chaos and violence, a senior British officer advised my grandfather to evacuate his own family to Gaza. My father very clearly recalls his father staying in Beersheba. He would later learn that his father imagined the situation to be temporary. He thought they would all be reunited in a couple of weeks to continue their lives in Beersheba. In the panic to leave, my grandmother, Yusra, wanted to take her sewing machine. However, her husband – thinking she could, of course, fetch it later – told her not to worry about it. Years later, Eyad would see his mother crying. She would cry over the loss of her beloved sewing machine. These notions of loss, dispossession and longing for return are a large part of the Palestinian story.

Oral testimonies collected by Rosemary Sayigh portray Palestinians pre-1948 as a community steeped in collective spirit with a profound sense of belonging. Their daily rituals of life provided enormous meaning and warmth. They had no idea of the imminent threat to their world:

> The last thing they were thinking of was to leave Palestine. Only a few young men who were educated realized at the end that their country was in danger. There was no consciousness. They lived daily — laughed, played, sang, went on outings. When young men and girls finished their work, they would search for a wedding to enjoy themselves. All was pleasure. They didn't see the difficulties of life. Few awakenings from 'unconsciousness' have been harsher or more abrupt.
>
> They had lived under many occupations, but none had ever displaced them from their land. They knew the Zionists aimed to possess Palestine, but they could not imagine a world in which such a thing could happen. Their belief in themselves, their ignorance of Zionist power (based on organization, not numbers), their old-fashioned concept of war, their naive dependence on Arab promises of help: all these prevented them from fully understanding what was happening in the 1940s, as Zionist preparations to take over the state mounted. [6]

This was a national trauma. It was a sudden loss without time to grieve or prepare. My father took that trip to Gaza as the second eldest, just four years old. He took that journey without his father, a source of protection and security. His mother demonstrated to Eyad who could look after and protect him. For much of this life, my father spoke about the importance of the father as a source of pride and as a protector. I can't help but wonder to what extent this early experience impacted his theories.

The Creation of the 'Gaza Strip'

The expression 'Gaza Strip' directly results from the changes caused by the *Nakba* in 1948. Zionist forces were ethnically cleansing large parts of Southern Palestine, forcing people to flee to what eventually became known as the Gaza Strip. This Zionist military plan, *Plan Dalet*, sought to remove Palestinians from their land and homes. In his famous book, historian Ilan Pappe details the massacres of these villages.[7] It was a horrifying time, and hoping to find safety, Palestinians fled to

Gaza's tiny strip of land. Egyptian forces attempted to protect Palestinians, and one Egyptian commander said:

> My military honour doesn't allow me to leave my Arab brothers and sisters, defenseless women and children, to be slaughtered by Jews like chicken.[8]

The Egyptian forces were able to defend Gaza, and the Gaza Strip was saved. Two hundred thousand refugees who had been depopulated from other parts of Palestine ended up in Gaza. By October 1948, Israel had expanded its control to 78% of British Mandated Palestinian territory. Of the original 900,000 – 950,000 Palestinians of the areas eventually incorporated into Israel, only 150,000 remained.[9] The rest had been expelled or fled to the West Bank, the Gaza Strip, or crossed into what became permanent refugee camps in Lebanon, Syria, and Jordan.

When you hear the term refugee, it conjures up negative images of an unwanted and desperate person. But the *Nakba* is a crucial reminder these people fleeing had homes, warmth, belonging and pride. They did not want to run. Instead, they were *made* into refugees, and 80 years later, these refugees are still reacting to the circumstances forced upon them. My father and his family were heading to Gaza, unaware that this was where they would be for the rest of their lives. They were unaware that 70 years later, Western political leaders would start referring to Gaza as a 'prison camp'.[10] Eyad had no idea that he would spend his life fighting for the rights of this community.

A New Reality

The influx of refugees to Gaza from all over Palestine had swelled the population of Gaza from 35,000 to 170,000. Initially, there was goodwill. The arriving Palestinians attempted to rent rooms, be housed in temporary public buildings, or even abandoned British army barracks. But it wasn't enough:

> People were forced to find shelter wherever they could: in huts without windows and often without roofs; in shelters made from branches and burlap bags; in caves; in orange groves; on sand dunes; and on the beaches, their houses made of blankets or palm branches draped around an old oar or mast stuck in the mud. Others lived in doorways and under the eaves of buildings. They filled the sidewalks, vacant lots, public markets, and barnyards-every available space. Asked what shelter they had, many refugees replied simply, 'the sky.'[11]

This desperation and suffering were to mark the beginning of the involvement of aid agencies in Palestine. Today it is a multi-billion-dollar global industry that has led to an enormous literature on aid, development, 'best practices' and exorbitant consultancy fees for internationals and staff.[12] However, in the beginning, there was a crisis. Aid agencies estimated that up to ten children were dying each day from hunger, cold and a lack of care. The United Nations Relief and Works Agency (UNRWA) was established in 1950 to address the growing number of desperate refugees. It still operates today. In a sign of global failure to address the systemic problems, 5 million refugees are now eligible for its services.[13]

One of the first agencies to work in Gaza, even before UNRWA, was the Quakers. The Quakers still exist today; their work grew out of Christianity, and while providing aid was necessary, so too was peace and reconciliation. They also believed in a practice known as 'bearing witness'. That expression was first said to me in 2009 by an activist in Gaza, and it didn't make much sense to me. However, it's a guiding theme of the Quakers' work, and I have noticed it's a philosophy of many visitors to Gaza. I now understand that bearing witness to something means one can go on to tell these stories to one's community. Therefore, it can help raise awareness, but it can also help change the individuals' values and beliefs.

In 1949, the Executive Secretary of the Quakers, Clarence E. Pickett, visited Palestine, including Gaza, for two months. He subsequently wrote an op-ed in the *Philadelphia Inquirer* titled 'Friends Feed Exiled Arabs':

> The relief program is well underway...This results in a ration of 2000 calories per day for each of the 200,000 refugees...We have distributed 1300 tents...We are also setting up a medical program...to head off epidemics.[14]

He then goes on to warn of the temporary nature of these programs:

> These services which I have described are definitely 'relief' services, hence temporary. Even if all the needs were taken care of, they would not be satisfied; they would still want to return to their homes and live their own lives.[15]

He presciently warns against failing to solve the 'refugee problem' a phrase that still echoes through the decades:

> To neglect this chance [resettlement] is to court future wars and retaliation for an indefinite time.[16]

To Mr Pickett, it was startlingly evident that this problem would not go away. Eyad once remarked that Palestinians would have been better off without UNRWA. He meant that the 'refugee problem' would have to have been dealt with. Instead, UNRWA has been given the responsibility of looking after refugees indefinitely. UNRWA's role in Palestine would become the centre of political negotiations and years of geopolitical conflict. In 2018 it even led to President Donald Trump revoking the US contribution to UNRWA's budget.[17]

Life in Gaza for Palestinians without homes was devastating. This catastrophic environment would shape the lives of Palestinians in Gaza, and their children, for generations. My father was 'lucky' as his grandfather already lived in Gaza. This meant that while they were refugees, they were not classified as refugees. I would later learn that this distinction is a source of status and pride in Gaza. UNRWA looked after refugees and provided a safety net. 'Original' Gazans, like my father's family, were not afforded refugee status, which meant they were not entitled to UNRWA welfare. Eyad also recalls the prejudice that emerged. For example, refugees and non-refugees were not supposed to marry, and mixing between the groups was not common. Although Eyad, with typical character, recalled having school friends from the camps.

On arrival in Gaza, Eyad recalls going straight to his grandfather's. They cowered in underground shelters as bombs dropped around them and the war for Palestine raged. With the view of one day settling in Gaza, Rajab, whilst in Beersheba, had been regularly sending money to build a home. After Eyad had spent critical time at their grandfather's, the family arrived at their new home in Remal. The house was small, but it had a veranda and a garden. Eyad's father found work quickly in UNRWA, which provided needed financial security.

Gaza's landscape was different to other parts of Palestine. There were no rolling hills like 'Southern Italy'. Instead, it was more desolate but retained much beauty, especially its views of the Mediterranean Sea. Rajab was a skilful and careful gardener, and in his spare time, grew a mini oasis. Over the following decades, my father took over his father's garden and continued to tend to it. It became a source of great calm and escape until his passing amidst the worsening political environment.

On May 15th, 1948, the State of Israel was proclaimed. Palestine had been transformed from a majority Arab country to a substantial Jewish majority. According to the historian Rashid Khalidi:

> This transformation was the result of two processes: the systematic ethnic cleansing of the Arab-inhabited areas of the country seized during the war; and the theft of Palestinian land and property left behind by the refugees as well as much of that owned by those Arabs who remained in Israel.[18]

A Violent Time

Despite the relative security that my grandfather enjoyed as a property owner and having an extended family in secure employment, Gaza was still a violent place. A new feature of life in Gaza was aerial bombings. Abu Sitta, in his memoir, describes them:

> The horror of the air raids was indescribable. People could not understand or predict when they would come. They could hear the roar of the approaching tanks. But air raids brought sudden, violent, and widespread death. You did not know when and from where the raids would come. You did not know whom they would hit. You could be killed but the person standing a few paces away might be safe. You could die at any moment. You could be out to get some food for your family and never come back....It was clear to us that the bombing was for the sole purpose of terrifying people and discouraging them from ever contemplating a return to their homes. There cannot have been a military reason for the bombing because the targets were all civilians. [19]

The Red Cross counted 227 corpses in one day of bombings, describing the scenes as unbelievable.[20] My father recalls hearing the bombs falling and being very frightened. The tragedy was that he would experience this again almost 60 years later during Operation Cast Lead in 2008.

In the 1950s, the UN and world leaders called for 'restraint from both sides' and made passive calls for de-escalation. In the 1950s, the UN was pleading with Israel, specifically Ben Gurion, to show restraint against Egypt's forces in Gaza:

> You [Ben Gurion] believe the threat of reprisals is a deterrent...You believe that reprisals will avoid future incidents. I believe that they will provoke future incidents. Dag Hammarskjold, UN Secretary-General[21]

The UN calls for restraint have been reverberating through the decades. And cycles of violence – which are typically a reference to discrete periods – are decades-long. So understanding today's violence in Gaza makes far more sense when looked at in historical context and through the lens of dispossession.

> On an almost monthly basis, Israelis raided the camps, killing and wounding people while they slept. It was no comfort to them that blue-eyed, blue-helmeted United Nations (UN) officers came, took notes and photographs, counted the dead, and then left. [22]

The refugees had been abandoned and did not feel protected by anyone. The tragedy of the bombings, and the UN reporting, is that they keep happening. It's not that the UN's words and report writing aren't necessary. What is hard to bear is the feeling of powerlessness as 60 years later, you see the same violence and the same toothless international reaction.

The First Occupation of Gaza

Gaza, since the *Nakba*, had been under the control of the Egyptians. At this time, Egypt was led by Nasser, the charismatic socialist leader and President of Egypt, who himself had fought in Gaza as an army officer. He was a hero to many in the Arab world. He espoused a vision of all Arabs as one people. A political idea that becomes known as Pan-Arabism. Nasser became a hero to many, becoming a source of pride and dignity. My grandfather was a big fan of Nasser's. Eyad's younger brother was named after Nasser.

Nasser's popularity soared when he nationalized the Suez Canal. It was seen as an attack on British, Israel and French forces, who had been colonizing parts of the region for centuries. A leader like Nasser offered a restoration of dignity and agency through his willingness to stand up physically to these colonial enemies.

However, one of the consequences of this was the likelihood of more violence – and from much more powerful forces. In October 1956, the leaders of France, Britain, and Israel launched an attack against Egypt. By November, the Israelis were firing artillery and air bombing the Gaza Strip. It was not long before Gaza was under Israeli control. Once Israel had taken control, the population were warned to stay at home via roving vehicles with public speakers. You can imagine eerie streets and terrified residents. This was the first occupation of Gaza by Israeli forces.

The occupation led to the rounding up and massacres of Palestinians in Gaza. There were two notable massacres of civilians. First, in the south of Gaza, a place called Khan Yunis. Palestinians were lined up against an old Ottoman wall and shot. The second was in a refugee camp, where approximately 415 people were killed. According to reports, the dead bodies were left out for days before families could collect them. One of the camp's residents was an eight-year-old boy named Abdel Aziz Ali Abdul Majid al-Rantissi.[23] Rantissi would go on to become the co-founder and leader of Hamas.

This violent episode is a stark reminder of the generational impact of violence on the Palestinian community. These stories of massacres passed down from one generation to the next are perhaps why my father's capacity for empathy, and not revenge, is so often spoken of as almost an aberration.[24]

As violence continued across Gaza, Eyad vividly recalls seeing the dead bodies of Egyptian soldiers strewn across the road.[25] His father refused to let him leave the house. Almost 60 years later, during the 2012 bombings, this is precisely how my father treated me. He refused to let us go near windows or doors. It was unthinkable to look out the window or go on the roof to get a better view. These were things that could get you killed.

During the Israeli occupation, Eyad was confined to his home and could only hear the loudspeaker announcements from the Israelis. One day, over this loudspeaker, he remembered a voice commanding all males over 18 to go to the Palestine School. Their justification was looking for *fedayeen* (Palestinian fighters). But the Israeli army was not discriminate: they rounded up people who simply had posters of Nasser on their walls.[26] The Israeli soldiers marched into Eyad's home, who at the time was 11. The soldier prodded his gun in between my father's shoulder blades. And a frightened Eyad reportedly wet himself.[27] I was never able to discuss this event with my father. However, what is clear is that he was growing up in a violent and uncertain environment—one which would seemingly offer a young Eyad little room to extend much compassion or empathy towards Israel.

By March 1957, the occupation had ended. The Israelis had left. The occupation of Gaza had ended because it was opposed by the new US President, Eisenhower. The US wanted Israel to end its occupation, and Ben Gurion, the Israeli Prime Minister, eventually agreed. The US felt that the conflict could lead to an opening for the Soviets, and Ben Gurion felt that there was no security benefit to occupying Gaza.[28] This event highlights the significant role the US would have over Israel and Palestine. Eyad would often say that the US would 'green light' operations on Gaza. He was right that the US wielded significant power over Israel. However, the actions of the US over multiple administrations suggest they rarely wielded their power to benefit Palestinians.

Coexistence

In the aftermath of the fighting, Eyad opened the door to a man who told him his name was Moshe. Moshe had come to visit Eyad's father. The presence of this Jewish man alarmed Eyad. Eyad discussed this experience in an interview with Terry Gross on *NPR's Fresh Air* and said that having never met a Jew, he – up until this point – had equated Jews with evil 'monsters'.[29] In front of Eyad, Moshe and Eyad's father embraced warmly. His father would later tell Eyad that Jews and Palestinians had been living side by side. He learned that it was Zionism and European Jewish migration that bought a different and more destructive ideology to Palestine.[30] As historians have noted, a large proportion of Jews living in Palestine in the first decade of the 20th Century were non-Zionist, Mizrahi (eastern) or Sephardic (Spain), urbanites of Middle Eastern origin or Mediterranean origin who often spoke Arabic or Turkish.[31]

It's hard to know how this event shaped Eyad's life. Many factors in my father's life would have shaped his future. Learning that Jews and Palestinians had co-existed was important. But what would have happened if he had witnessed the massacres in camps like Rantissi had? Would he have been less forgiving? Stories of a peaceful co-existence between Jews and Palestinians can offer a bulwark against the trauma of violence and dehumanizing language. Despite these stories of coexistence, Israeli leaders were well aware of the hatred they were sowing:

> Why should we complain about their burning hatred for us? For eight years they have been sitting in the refugee camps in Gaza, watching us transforming the lands and the villages where they and their fathers dwelt, into our property—Moshe Dayan, 1956[32]

With hatred being nourished in Gaza by Israel's policies, not everyone wanted to choose the path of coexistence. Ramzy Baroud details his father's reaction:

> Mohammed saw in the Fedayeen and their stories a heroic escape from his humiliating life. As envious as he was of his older brother, he no longer fantasized about being a teacher. Freedom fighting became his new calling. The Fedayeen were the antithesis to his humiliation and submissiveness, and a manifestation of all the anger and frustration he felt. He wanted to go back to Beit Daras so badly that he would constantly investigate whether any of the commandos passed by his village, or had a glimpse of his old school by the hill. He offered his services as a watchman for the Fedayeen as they made their initial, and most dangerous, crossovers into Israel. He would try to impress his family with his bravery. They ridiculed his active imagination and asked him to keep his focus on selling his knick-knacks. But Mohammed was adamant that he would join a resistance group as soon as it was possible. [33]

The two stories of Eyad and Ramzy Baroud's father offer two distinct experiences. All Palestinians are dealing with humiliation, the loss of their father as a source of protection, and exposure to violence and death. How each Palestinian deals with these psychological wounds will vary. Eyad wrote:

> Children are conscious of the fact that their fathers cannot protect them. The trauma they have experienced has led to a state of emotional detachment. They are talking to you as if it happened to someone else. There is a suppression of pain – they cannot integrate their experience into their personality. Over the short-term Post Traumatic Stress Disorder will develop

in the children. The long-term effects will be felt in the next generation, also because of children responding to their parents' behaviour.[34]

The psychological wounds of the *Nakba* had been inflicted on two generations. Over the next 60 years, Palestinians would have to cope with the events of the *Nakba* and much more violence and loss. Eyad felt the agony of Gaza deeply and would spend his life trying to heal these wounds.

Notes

1. Baroud, R 2009, *My Father Was a Freedom Fighter: Gaza's Untold Story*, Pluto Press, London, pp14
2. Kardahji, N 2007, *A Measure of Restraint: The Palestine Police and the End of the British Mandate*, MPhil Thesis, Oxford University, Oxford, England.
3. Filiu, J 2014, *Gaza: A History*, Hurst & Company, London, pp53
4. Khalidi, R 2020, *The Hundred Years' War on Palestine: A History of Settler Colonialism and Resistance, 1917–2017*, Metropolitan Books, New York, pp60
5. Black, I 2018, *Enemies and Neighbours: Arabs and Jews in Palestine and Israel, 1917-2017*, Penguin, London, pp201
6. Sayigh, R 1979, *Palestinians: From Peasants to Revolutionaries*, Zed Books, London, pp4
7. Pappe, I 2007, *The Ethnic Cleansing of Palestine*, One World, London
8. Souri, H 2016, *Gaza as Metaphor*, Hurst, London, pp105
9. Younes, A 2020, 'Nakba Day: For Palestinians, not just an historical event', *Al Jazeera Online*, May 15th
10. Watt, N 2010, David Cameron: Israeli blockade has turned Gaza Strip into a 'prison camp', *Guardian*, 27th July
11. Cheal, B 1988, 'Refugees in the Gaza Strip December 1948-May 1950', *Journal of Palestine Studies*, Vol18 (1), Autumn, pp. 138-157
12. Taghdisi-Rad, S 2015, *The Political Economy of Aid in Palestine Relief from Conflict or Development Delayed?*, Routledge, UK
13. https://www.unrwa.org/palestine-refugees
14. Pickett, C 1949, 'Friends Feed Exiled Arabs', *Philadelphia Enquirer*, March 20th
15. ibid
16. ibid
17. Amr, H 2018, 'In one move, Trump eliminated US funding for UNRWA and the US role as Mideast peacemaker', *Brookings*, September 7th
18. Khalidi, R 2020, *The Hundred Years' War on Palestine: A History of Settler Colonialism and*

Resistance, 1917–2017, Metropolitan Books, New York, pp75

19. Abu Sitta, S 2016, *Mapping My Return: A Palestinian Memoir*, The American University in Cairo Press, Cairo, pp86
20. Abu Sitta, S 2016, *Mapping My Return: A Palestinian Memoir*, The American University in Cairo Press, Cairo, pp86
21. Baconi, T 2018, 'What the Gaza Protests Portend', *New York Review of Books*, May 15th
22. Abu Sitta, S 2016, *Mapping My Return: A Palestinian Memoir*, The American University in Cairo Press, Cairo, pp104
23. Filiu, J 2014, *Gaza: A History*, Hurst & Company, London, pp97
24. *National Public Radio* (NPR) 2001, 'Fresh Air Archive: Interviews with Terry Gross. Eyad El-Sarraj', <https://freshairarchive.org/segments/eyad-el-sarraj> [Accessed 1 October 2021].
25. Aaron, P 2016, 'The Pathological Optimist: One Man's Vision for Palestinian Well-Being', *Journal of Palestine Studies*, V45(2
26. Filiu, J 2014, *Gaza: A History*, Hurst & Company, London, pp98
27. Aaron, P 2016, 'The Pathological Optimist: One Man's Vision for Palestinian Well-Being', *Journal of Palestine Studies*, V45(2)
28. Filiu, J 2014, *Gaza: A History*, Hurst & Company, London, pp103
29. *National Public Radio* (NPR) 2001, 'Fresh Air Archive: Interviews with Terry Gross. 2021. Eyad El-Sarraj' <https://freshairarchive.org/segments/eyad-el-sarraj> [Accessed 1 October 2021].
30. ibid
31. Khalidi, R 2020, *The Hundred Years' War on Palestine: A History of Settler Colonialism and Resistance, 1917–2017*, Metropolitan Books, New York, pp19
32. *Jewish Virtual Library* 1956, Moshe Dayan's Eulogy for Roi Rutenberg - April 19, viewed online August 21st 2020 <https://www.jewishvirtuallibrary.org/moshe-dayans-eulogy-for-roi-rutenberg-april-19-1956>
33. Baroud, R 2009, *My Father Was a Freedom Fighter: Gaza's Untold Story*, Pluto Press, London, pp47
34. Jasiewicz, E 2015, 'I saw a man beheaded', *Red Pepper*, December 10th

4. EGYPT: COLLECTIVE JOY

A strong, free call came up from the people. A voice that is independent, strong and deep, Saying: 'I am the people, I am the miracle.' I am the people, nothing can stop me, And everything I say I do. —Um Kulthum, *On the Gates to Egypt*

I recently attended a comedy event in London: the Egyptian/American comedian told her audience that she had recently performed in Palestine. She retold a moment from being on stage in Palestine: 'My parents wanted me to be a doctor or an engineer, but I ended up being a comedian...'. But before completing the joke, a Palestinian man in her Palestinian audience, with sincerity, said: 'It's ok habibti (my love), you still have time but only if you work hard.'

The joke of the well-meaning parent wanting their child to be a doctor or an engineer but not paying sufficient attention to the child's 'true calling', is well known. My father was to be no exception. He had always wanted to be a farmer or work outdoors on land. His mother, with practical wisdom, amended his application for the university to 'Medicine'. Education was a precious commodity for Palestinians, and many hoped that their children would earn enough to support the whole family.

Nasser, in Egypt, was riding a wave of popularity and sent a powerful message to Palestinians when he announced free education for Palestinians who chose to study in Egypt. Under Nasser, Egypt was to become a mecca for poor Palestinian students. Instead, Palestinians ended up in big cities like Alexandria or Cairo. Abu Sitta recounts moving to Cairo with his brothers to continue his school education. They went from educated Palestinian notables to being perceived by Egyptians as refugee criminals.[1] It was a humiliating and challenging transition for many to make.

However, some joy and dignity were to come in the form of the Palestinian Students' Union (PSU). The PSU was created in Cairo and was a democratic vehicle that sought to give voice to Palestinians. Eyad would eventually join it, and it turns out many Palestinians were interested in the lure of the PSU. This was because these young, passionate students, whose families were suffering, who were at the mercy of Israel's power, could not organise in the West Bank or Jordan. In this context, in 1962, Eyad moved to Alexandria to take up his studies, and an entirely new world of energised, young Palestinian revolutionaries awaited him.

When I interviewed Salam Fayyad, the former Prime Minister of the Palestinian Authority and longtime friend of Eyad's, he described Eyad as an 'artist'. Of course, he was not talking about paint. But he was describing a man who was creative and connected to humans at a deep emotional level. It was no surprise then that this proclivity meant he was mainly unsuited to the rote learning of studying medicine. I remember him telling me how he hated learning so many 'boring' Latin words.

I never saw the disciplined academic in my father, who spends hours toiling away on their own – perhaps others did. But to me, he was more social and spontaneous. He told me he 'loved' to be around people, and it almost didn't matter who he was with. He loved the energy, and I think this socialising habit helped make him an astute observer of human behaviour. It also provided ample practice to tell stories – something he was especially good at.

In Alexandria, Eyad's interest in psychiatry was perhaps partially triggered by his experience with a roommate who tragically killed himself.[2] Upon completing his medical training, he told his supervisor that he was interested in psychology and philosophy. These are disciplines that, of course, are about humans but situate humans in a much richer context of their lived experience. It was natural for a medical student with such an interest to study psychiatry. His supervisor arranged for an internship in psychiatry at Cairo's Abbasiya Mental Hospital and Asylum. This was a vast complex and the largest institution of its kind in the Middle East. An appalled Eyad witnessed doctors and nurses treat patients with indifference. He would watch and think to himself why nobody listened to the patients. He could not understand why they were not treated with more compassion, more dignity.[3]

When I learned how my father felt during his time on a psychiatric ward, it offered a moment of reflection. I had worked as a healthcare assistant in a psychiatric ward in North London. It was my first job in mental health too. I ended up writing about my experiences online for the *Guardian*.[4] I made almost identical observations that my father had completed 50 years prior. I watched patients treated like numbers, left to their distress alone, and drugged to be kept at bay. But what was so obvious was the lack of dignity and compassion with which they were so often treated.

All the violence and shouting I witnessed was almost always a consequence of a perceived lack of dignity or freedom. The patients wanted to phone a loved one to reclaim possession of theirs. The indifference that nurses would show, or lack of attention, would only further frustrate the patient. Their lashing out was often distress. It was, in some cases, the build-up of a lifetime of not having their 'needs met' and of being neglected. The parallels with Palestinians, with Gaza, are clear. Eyad's observations on the psychiatric wards of the role of dignity, fairness and freedom would become some of his guiding principles.

Radical Happiness

It's no surprise that my father spent his time in Alexandria, preferring to socialise and talk about politics. The difference between that time and now is just how politically charged and – crucially – hopeful the environment was. These were exciting times, and the lure of politics was not just about 'virtue signalling' or getting 'likes' on social media; it was about undertaking actions with the explicit, urgent and immediate aim of freeing your homeland – your family – from occupation. He was at the centre of change and surrounded by his kindred brothers. Arguably it was this feeling of radical collectivism and purpose from which my father could never turn away.

As an example of just how electrifying the environment was, Nasser had become the icon of something called the 'non-aligned' movement. His star power attracted many people to the region, including Gaza. The likes of Malcolm X and Che Guevara were all seen photographed in Gaza.[5] The following is a description of Malcolm X's trip to Gaza:

> After the summit ended, Malcolm embarked on a two-day trip to Gaza on September 4, 1964. After checking in to the Kuwait Hotel along the Mediterranean Sea, he spent some time shopping in town in as much as the Egyptians had declared Gaza a duty-free zone and many products were available in the markets there that could not be found back in Egypt.
>
> The next day, he met with the Egyptian assistant military governor of Gaza, Colonel Mustafa Khafaja, and visited several Palestinian refugee camps, a hospital, and the area along the cease-fire lines with Israel. He also lunched with some Islamic religious leaders and heard about Israel's brief 1956–57 invasion and occupation of Gaza from an eyewitness, a man named Harun Hashim Rashid.
>
> Malcolm also held a press conference at the Palestinian Legislative Council building in Gaza City. Topping off a long day, he performed evening prayers at a mosque along with the mayor of Gaza City, Munir al-Rayyis. He returned to Cairo the following day, September 6.[6]

What is interesting about this trip is the nature of global solidarity – which has echoes of black liberation movements – and the role that visiting international figures were starting to play. When I was in Gaza from 2009-2012, I was privy to many people visiting Gaza, such as Jimmy Carter, US Congressman Keith Ellison, Noam Chomsky, and Naomi Klein. They all paid a visit to Eyad in the hope he could help them understand more about Gaza. There is no doubt that if Eyad was hosting political salons in the 1960s, Malcolm X would have visited him.

Of course, the visitors to Palestine, like Malcolm X, come with different motivations, but there is an importance to internationals visiting Palestine. Firstly, reporting back to their community is important, which echoes the notion of bearing witness that the Quakers pioneered. There is also an opportunity to build links between institutions inside and outside Gaza. Bringing Gaza to the world was at the core of my father's work. He knew that nurturing solidarity, materially and emotionally, could be an essential factor for political change.

Eyad's political life started when he was elected head of Alexandria's Palestinian Students' Union (PSU). One of his early challenges was to get his bloc enough seats in an upcoming election. A friend of Eyad's from that period recalls seeing the poster he had designed, which – unusually – contained a poem from Mahmoud Darwish, with the lines:

> *My country is not a suitcase*
> *I am not a traveler*
> *I am the lover and the land is the beloved.*[7]

The poster was emotionally evocative and conveyed how much of Eyad's soul was wrapped up in his politics. He also found that he was adept at talking to people and convincing them to vote. Charm was often said to be something my father had. I think charm is too loose an expression, as charisma is often associated with politicians who sell empty promises. I think what my father had was a sincere belief that he was acting in pursuit of justice. It is this belief, this confident sense of purpose, which can be incredibly captivating.

It was not long before Eyad was elected as vice-president of the international organisation of the General Union of Palestinian Students (GUPS). The GUPS had been the first democratically elected Palestinian organisation, and its precursor, the Palestinian Students Union (PSU) in Cairo, provided a representative voice for Palestinians.[8] The GUPS was the centre of political activity for Palestinians in the diaspora. The GUPS was delivering the first opportunity for Palestinians in the diaspora to come together, engage each other, and develop a common Palestinian identity. Indeed, the GUPS was the first to call for the establishment of a Palestinian entity, a liberation army, and a liberation organisation. And it was from this group of young students that the future leaders of the Palestinian movement would come. Most famously Yasser Arafat was president between 1952-1956.

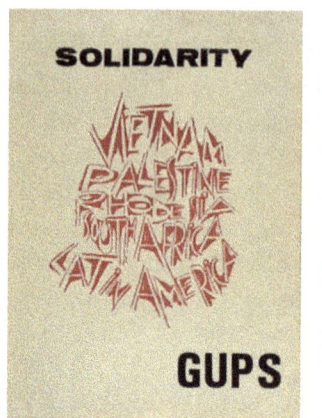 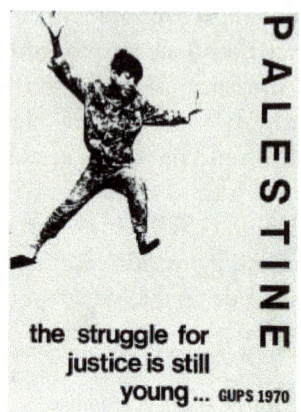

Posters Published by GUPS, 1970

During this period, different groups were emerging claiming to speak for Palestinians. In 1964 the Palestine Liberation Organisation (PLO) was established by Egypt. Its first head was Ahmed Shukeiri, with whom Eyad would become friends. Tension soon emerged between the democratic GUPS and the PLO. The PLO had indicated the GUPS was in some way its political base. But the GUPS issued a rebuttal in order to stake its independence. Over time, Arafat and Fatah consolidated control of the PLO.

Eyad had been in Nasser's Egypt at a critical period. Under Nasser, Palestinians from Gaza and elsewhere had been able to lay down the groundwork for a national movement. This period politicised an entire generation. However, despite Eyad's success at student elections and being courted by Fatah and the PLO representatives, he stayed away from tribal politics. He valued critical thinking and curiosity, and his moral values could not be compromised. However, in Cairo, he got a taste of political organising that never left him and informed much of his work.

Permission to Narrate

In 1967 Egypt went to war with Israel and lost. In six days, Israel seized the remaining Palestinian territories of the West Bank, East Jerusalem and the Gaza Strip, the Syrian Golan Heights and the Egyptian Sinai Peninsula.[9] Palestinians refer to this as the *Naksa*: 'a return to 1967 borders' means a return to the land lost during this war.

In response, the UN developed resolution 242.[10] According to Arafat, who was now the leader of the PLO, the 1967 defeat was a 'great incentive for us'.[11] His statements reflected the failure of the Arab states to defeat Israel. In losing so heavily, Arafat was able to reframe the struggle for Palestine. Instead of relying on Arab states to rescue them, they would now be able to put forward their own ideas of resistance, namely that armed struggle was central to achieving freedom for the Palestinians.

Globally, Arafat was becoming well known, even appearing on the cover of *Time Magazine*. On Arafat's popularity and the rise of Arafat's PLO, Eyad reflected: '…people did not know what Palestinian identity was at this point until Arafat took over the PLO. He embodied our national identity.'[12]

When Arafat died, I remember my father crying. He told me it wasn't so much mourning about his character as much as the meaning and the tragedy of his loss. It felt to me like these were all men from the same generation trying to help Palestinians. They, of course, disagreed fiercely with the methods and strategy. However, there was still this feeling, not unquestioned loyalty, but certainly, solidarity between each other, which was meaningful to my father and many more Palestinians.

Notes

1. Abu Sitta, S 2016, *Mapping My Return: A Palestinian Memoir*, The American University in Cairo Press, Cairo, pp76
2. Aaron, P 2016, 'The Pathological Optimist: One Man's Vision for Palestinian Well-Being', *Journal of Palestine Studies*, V45(2)
3. Ibid
4. Sarraj, W 2015, 'We healthcare assistants are the least trained but most hands-on NHS staff', *The Guardian*, March 12th, <https://www.theguardian.com/healthcare-network/2015/mar/12/healthcare-assistant-nhs-mental-health-patients>
5. Filiu, J 2014, *Gaza: A History*, Hurst & Company, London, pp131
6. Fishbach, M 2018, *Black Power and Palestine: Transnational Countries of Color*, Stanford University Press, US
7. Darwish, M, 'Diary of a Palestinian Wound', Available online at: <https://www.arabicnadwah.com/arabicpoetry/darwish-diary.htm>
8. Brand, L 1988, 'Nasir's Egypt and the Reemergence of the Palestinian National Movement', *Journal of Palestine Studies*, Vol. 17, No. 2 (Winter), pp. 29-45
9. Al Tahhan, Z 2018, 'The Naksa: How Israel occupied the whole of Palestine in 1967', *Al Jazeera*, June 4th
10. UN, Resolution 242 (1967) of 22 November 1967, Available online at: <https://unis-

pal.un.org/unispal.nsf/0/7d35e1f729df491c85256ee700686136>/footnote] The resolution meant Israel would only need to withdraw from these newly conquered territories if it negotiated with the neighbouring Arab states. UN resolution 242 was supported by the British and Americans. In this context, Palestine was not mentioned, so, in effect, Palestinians didn't exist. Palestinians were considered more of a refugee and humanitarian problem. Resolution 242 also glossed over the loss of land in 1948. From now onwards, the world saw the borders of 1967 as the new starting point for negotiations.[footnote]Khalidi, R 2020, *The Hundred Years' War on Palestine: A History of Settler Colonialism and Resistance, 1917–2017*, Metropolitan Books, New York, pp106

11. Al Jazeera 2009, 'PLO, History of a Revolution: Intifada', <https://www.aljazeera.com/program/plo-history-of-a-revolution/2009/8/16/plo-history-of-a-revolution-intifada>

12. Neslen, A 2011, *In Your Eyes a Sandstorm. Ways of Being Palestinian*, University of California Press, US, pp255

5. RETURNING TO GAZA

> *[Gaza] equals the history of an entire homeland, because it is more ugly, impoverished, miserable, and vicious in the eyes of enemies. Because it is the most capable, among us, of disturbing the enemy's mood and his comfort. Because it is his nightmare. Because it is mined oranges, children without a childhood, old men without old age and women without desires. Because of all this it is the most beautiful, the purest and richest among us and the one most worthy of love.* —Mahmoud Darwish, *Silence for Gaza*

In the years before Eyad's return to Gaza in 1971, Ariel Sharon, Israel's military commander and future Prime Minister led a brutal crackdown on Gaza's Palestinian resistance. During this period, various factions were attempting to resist Israel's occupation. The Popular Front for the Liberation of Palestine (PFLP), a Marxist-Leninist and revolutionary socialist-inspired group, was launching attacks. The PFLP's Muhammad al-Aswad, nicknamed 'Guevara of Gaza', had become legendary in leading efforts against the Israeli forces.[1] Arafat's Fatah and George Habash's PFLP were to become the two dominant resistance factions.

In the first half of 1970, 352 armed operations against Israel in Gaza were claimed to have been conducted. In that year, there were 17 Israeli deaths, including eight soldiers, and 109 wounded. There were 110 Palestinian deaths and 667 wounded.[2] At this time, Israel also continued to use collective punishment and exile Palestinian civilians. Six hundred women and children were sent to a camp in the Sinai owing to their affiliations with resistance fighters.[3]

Jordan attempted to root out and end Palestinian operations initiated in Jordan. This led to massacres in Palestinian camps, in a period known famously as 'Black September'.[4] The combined efforts of Jordanian and Israeli forces proved too much, and the *fedayeen* (Palestinian fighters) were defeated. The Palestinian resistance leadership had been basing itself in supportive Arab countries such as Jordan and Egypt until this point. However, now they were exiled from Jordan, and their other ally, Nasser, died in September 1970. The PLO, under Arafat, from a position of weakness, would be increasingly forced to take things into their own hands. They had started to consider creating their own state alongside Israel in what became known as the 'two-state solution'.

'Dr Eyad'

Eyad's political consciousness had formed during Nasser's era, a period whose generation has been described as 'Nasser's Children'.[5] With these powerful experiences of political organizing, he left Cairo as both an educated man and a political activist. However, there was intense pressure and expectation on him to work and support his family. The Gaza people's access to a relatively good education in Egyptian universities and the Gulf States' need for teachers, doctors, and other professions made Palestinians the most suitable candidates for a range of jobs.[6] Indeed, my father turned down jobs in the Gulf. However, he eventually responded to a call from the International Committee of the Red Cross (ICRC).

The ICRC was established in 1863. It's described as: '...*an independent, neutral organization ensuring humanitarian protection and assistance for victims of war and armed violence. It takes action in response to emergencies and promotes respect for international humanitarian law and its implementation in national law.*[7]

The original call Eyad responded to is referenced in the 1971 annual report:[8]

STUDY OF HEALTH SITUATION ON THE GOLAN HEIGHTS, IN GAZA AND SINAI

"In March 1971, an ICRC doctor-delegate made a survey of the medical situation on the Golan Heights. In August, two similar surveys were conducted in the Gaza Strip and in Sinai, where all government and private hospitals and dispensaries were visited. Comprehensive reports were sent to the governments concerned.

In the course of an operation carried out under ICRC auspices at El Quantara, on 17 November, eleven doctors, who had originally come from Gaza and were living in Cairo, crossed the Suez Canal from west to east to resume work in the Gaza Strip, where a serious dearth of medical personnel was still prevailing."

Eyad had left Gaza occupied by Egypt, and he returned to his beloved Gaza under the next iteration of foreign control: Israel's violent occupation. The occupation wasn't only a military presence. Israel was directly controlling the civil servants in the health, education, and social services departments. Health, of course, is the department in which Eyad would be working. Navigating this hostile landscape, Eyad had to adjust to the violence and the lack of control over his own life. He also had to deal with a Gaza with his mother gone and his father now remarried. Despite this, he was still surrounded by loving family and dear friends. He often spoke about how sustaining they were for him.

Young but politically savvy from his time in Cairo and one of only 27 doctors in the entire Gaza Strip, he started work in the Pediatric Department at Shifa Hospital. Shifa Hospital, meaning 'house of healing' in Arabic, still exists today. It was originally established during the British Mandate. It's where I took a family member to have stitches removed in 2010, and it is where international medical staff often perform free surgeries.

Under Israeli occupation in the 1970s, Eyad had to report to Israeli intelligence so that he could get his ID and paperwork, a method of Israeli control that I also had to carry out in 2006. In 1971 the Israeli intelligence asked Eyad many questions about his time in Cairo. They were trying to gauge his level of political activism. This tense meeting ended with the Israeli officer asking him to write down all the names of his professors in Cairo. Confused and apprehensive, Eyad took some time to realize he was being asked to collaborate. Sticking to his gut feeling, he decided not to see this officer again, instead choosing to carry on working.[9]

It was not long before his Palestinian manager handed him a letter. The Israeli officer stated that for security reasons, Eyad was no longer allowed to work at the hospital. His refusal to collaborate had irked the Israelis. Undeterred, Eyad's innate sense of justice and courage kicked in. Within weeks, he mobilized other doctors to sign a petition, contacted the WHO and the head of the church in Gaza, and distributed a public statement. He was reinstated. His time in Cairo had taught him about political activism and the role of media advocacy. This was a set of skills he would use to great effect throughout his life.

In the early 1970s, Palestine was capturing the world's attention. To achieve this media coverage, parts of the PLO and PFLP had decided to use attention-grabbing tactics. The Black September Group emerged out of tactical disagreements within Fatah. Black September viewed getting media attention through public spectacles (often violent) as a viable tactic. To this end, they held Israeli Olympians hostage at the 1972 Munich Olympic Games; two Israeli athletes were killed. According to US cables, they also executed the American ambassador to Sudan, which was carried out with Arafat's knowledge.[10] By the end of 1973, the PLO leaders decided that Black September had served its purpose. Such attention was no longer helpful, as Arafat shifted to pursue diplomatic means.

The PFLP were infamously engaged in plane hijackings. The female resistance fighter Leila Khaled would become the face of these hijackings. Responding to accusations of violence and the hurting of innocent civilians, Leila says she was under strict instructions not to hurt anyone. And after three plane hijackings, nobody was hurt; they were 'clean', she says.¹¹ Despite the no harm policy, Palestinians were being portrayed globally as 'terrorists', and many felt this was counterproductive.

Bedlam

The only major mental health facility in Palestine was the Bethlehem Government Hospital, directed by a Maudsley-trained Palestinian psychiatrist, Mohamed Said Kamal. In 1993 the hospital was renamed in Dr Kamal's honour.¹² This was the obvious choice for Eyad to pursue further psychiatric training. Eyad worked at the hospital in 1972 and stayed there for approximately 18 months.

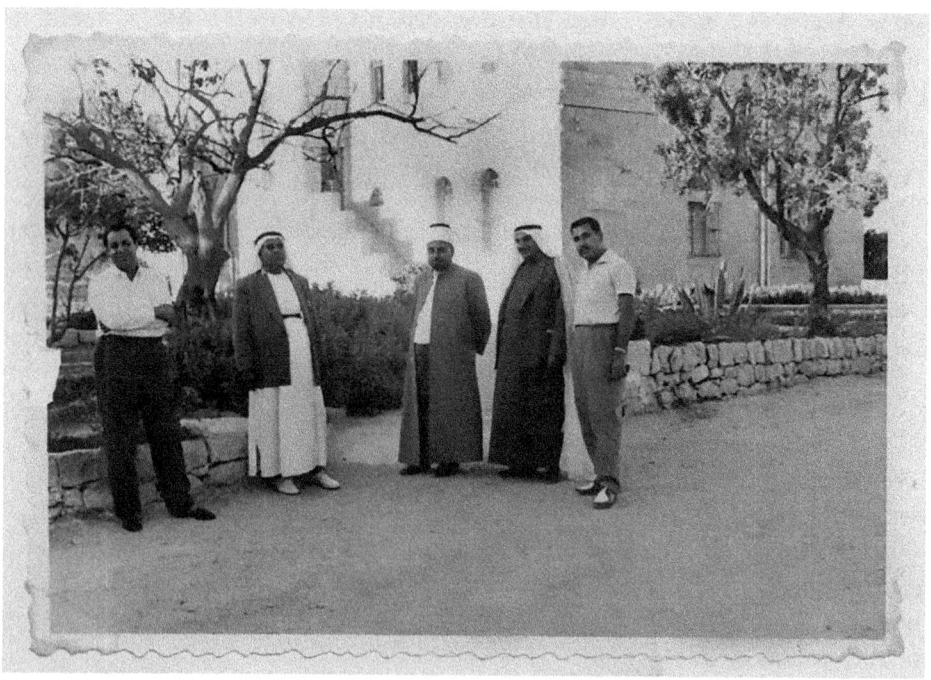

Men in front of the Mental Health Hospital, Bethlehem, 1958

Here, Eyad learned much about treating acutely ill patients. However, at that time, the acutely ill, such as those experiencing depression and diagnosed with schizophrenia, were being treated with electroconvulsive therapy. This left little room for learning other methods of treating those in distress. It wasn't until 1974 that the first community mental health clinic opened in the West Bank. Eyad's time in Bethlehem ended before the new community clinics were opened. He was about to embark on a new chapter, as he had been lucky enough to receive a scholarship, like a hospital's own director, to train at the world-famous Maudsley Hospital in London.

As my father touches down in London, Arafat is receiving a standing ovation at the United Nations General Assembly (UNGA). The fourth war between Israel and Arab states in 1973, known as the Yom Kippur war, ushered in a new political landscape. It had revealed the limits of what collective action by Arab allies of Palestine could achieve. Arafat was also convinced that the violence carried out by Black September had only harmed the reputation of the Palestinians abroad. Arafat had gone from 'commando' featured on the cover of *Time Magazine* to become a diplomat. His speech at the UN, drafted by Palestinian intellectual, Edward Said, is etched into history:

> "Today I have come bearing an olive branch and a freedom fighter's gun. Do not let the olive branch fall from my hand. I repeat: Do not let the olive branch fall from my hand." – Yasser Arafat, 1974, UNGA[13]

The UN responded with a standing ovation. Arafat's plea to the United Nations-led to the PLO being granted Observer Status, and their right to self-determination was granted. This was a significant moment, given that the UN and the other great powers had not recognized Palestine until this point. Moreover, Arafat and the PLO were having diplomatic success in the United National General Assembly. But, of course, Israel still had the upper hand, and the PLO had much work to do if they wanted to take advantage of these hard-won opportunities.

With the *fedayeen* defeated, who had been a major political force, opportunities emerged for other political ideas and institutions to emerge. For example, in 1973, Sheikh Yassin, a paralyzed Islamic Sheikh from Gaza, opened a mosque (with Israel's support) that would help nurture Islamic piety that helped to draw people away from nationalism.[14] Later, in 1987, Sheikh Yassin would go on to found Hamas. But it was this act in 1973 that helped pave the way for Islamist politics in Gaza and would have significant consequences.

The political climate was changing. The PLO was now pushing for diplomatic recognition, and the world was starting to understand that there were many faces to the Palestinian struggle. So setting off to London, Eyad was about to be a Palestinian man in Britain. It's a new culture and with this comes not just how you see yourself but how others choose to see you. Would he be seen as an 'angry Arab'? A terrorist? A charming doctor?

Notes

1. Filiu, J 2014, *Gaza: A History*, Hurst & Company, London, pp141
2. Filiu, J 2014, *Gaza: A History*, Hurst & Company, London, pp140
3. Ibid
4. Wolf, J 1973, 'Black September: Militant Palestinianism', *Current History*, V64(377), pp5-8
5. Filiu, J 2014, *Gaza: A History*, Hurst & Company, London, pp107
6. Baroud, R 2009, *My Father Was a Freedom Fighter: Gaza's Untold Story*, Pluto Press, London, pp68
7. ICRC Website, Who We Are <https://www.icrc.org/en/who-we-are>
8. International Committee of the Red Cross 1971, *Annual report*, retrieved from <https://library.icrc.org/library/search/notice?noticeNr=31083>
9. Aaron, P 2016, 'The Pathological Optimist: One Man's Vision for Palestinian Well-Being', *Journal of Palestine Studies*, V45(2)
10. Al Jazeera 2009, 'PLO, History of a Revolution: Intifada', <https://www.aljazeera.com/program/plo-history-of-a-revolution/2009/8/16/plo-history-of-a-revolution-intifada>
11. Neslen, A. 2011, *In Your Eyes a Sandstorm. Ways of Being Palestinian*, University of California Press, US, pp204
12. Al-Istiqlal University, 2017, 'The Students of Psychology Department Visit the Psychiatric Hospital in Bethlehem'
13. Shatz, A 2021, 'Palestinianism', *London Review of Books*, Vol. 43 No. 9, 6th May
14. Filiu, J 2014, *Gaza: A History*, Hurst & Company, London, pp159

6. LONDON

> **Lord Wigg:** My Lords, is the noble Lord aware that the terrorist activities of the Palestine Liberation Organisation, which all civilised men deplore, have their origin in the similar activities of the Irgun Zvei Leumi in Israel, many of whose members are now regarded as honoured citizens? Is not the lesson to be drawn from this that terrorist methods, if successful, lead to the terrorists being accepted as respectable members of society?
> **Lord Roberts:** My Lords, we all know that violence begets violence, and that this country condemns violence wherever it occurs.
> —Debate at the House of Lords on 'Palestine Liberation Organisation'
> —Volume 351: debated on Tuesday 14 May 1974, *Hansard Record*

The debate in the House of Lords reflected the growing attention acts of violence orchestrated by Palestinian factions were receiving. One of the triggers for this global upsurge in violence was Arafat and the PLO's decision to pursue diplomacy. This led to a rift within the Palestinian movement, with some labelling Arafat a 'sell-out'.[1] The PFLP, and a group headed by Abu Nidal, were at the centre of a range of methods that sought to capture the world's attention and undermine the nascent 'two-state solution'.

Perhaps most notorious was the work of the PFLP recruit 'Carlos the Jackal'. Carlos was a Venezuelan who worked with the PFLP to conduct assassinations and plane hijackings. One of his first missions took place in London in 1973. It was in St John's Wood, London, where he attempted to murder Joseph Sieff, president of the retailer Marks & Spencer (M&S) and honorary vice-president of the British Zionist Federation.[2] He burst into the St John's Wood mansion and demanded that Sieff's butler take him to Sieff. He opened fire and shot Sieff in the head. However, his gun jammed, he fled the scene, and Sieff survived. At the time, the PFLP were reported as saying the assassination attempt on Joseph Sieff was because he was playing 'host' to Israeli leader Menachem Begin.[3]

According to the *Birmingham Post*, prominent Jews feared being on a 'death list'.[4] The use of the term death list brings up horrifying symbolism from Nazi Germany. Although Abu Nidal's faction was nihilistically targeting Jews and Palestinians, they were deemed to have affiliations with Israel and Zionism.[5] It was a strategy that portrayed Palestinians as unhinged and murderous. The fear within Europe's Jewish community generated by this kind of violence and subsequent media portrayal is meaningful. The stories of these events that get repeated within communities can still play a role in current tensions over Israel, Palestine, Zionism, and antisemitism.

Assassinations were not only being carried out by Palestinians. Israel, too, was murdering not only political figures in Palestine but also its cultural figures. Ghassan Kanafani was a Palestinian refugee in Lebanon. He was a journalist, storyteller, activist and eventually spokesman for the PFLP. He was not involved in the PFLP's military wing nor the planning of any military resistance. He was multi-talented, and many felt that he could speak and write with unrivalled clarity that was able to cut through myths about Palestine, helping to communicate uncomfortable truths to the world.[6] Ghassan Kanafani was killed by an Israeli car bomb in 1972. Israel was seeking to stifle any Palestinian voices that sought to inspire and move their national movement.[7]

Amidst the violence and even attempts on Arafat's life, the PLO attempted to sow seeds for peace talks. Based in London was Said Hammami. He was the PLO's representative and was busy meeting diplomats and writing articles for publications such as *The Times*:

> Many Palestinians believe that a Palestinian state on the Gaza Strip and the West Bank, including al-Hammah region, is a necessary part of any peace package. Such a Palestinian state would lead to the emptying and closing down of the refugee camps, thereby drawing out the poison at the heart of Arab-Israeli enmity. It is no small thing for a people who have been wronged as we have to take the first step towards reconciliation for the sake of a just peace that should satisfy all parties.[8]

It was widely considered that Arafat and the PLO, through Hammami, were laying the groundwork for the 'two-state solution'. Uri Avnery, the notable Israeli peace activist, met Hammami and, according to him, Hammami was the first PLO representative to meet an Israeli intentionally.[9] There was real fear in the air at that time. Palestinians were killing other Palestinians, who were deemed to be capitulating, and the Israeli secret service (Mossad) was killing PLO officials. Even my father recalled being worried about secret police overhearing political conversations.

Paranoia was everywhere. Learning that Avnery was meeting the PLO in London in 1974 is remarkable: not the event itself, but the connection with my father's life. I was copied on emails that Avnery was sending to Eyad in 2012. They were trying to establish dialogue for reconciliation. Avnery's long commitment to peace is extraordinary and much has been written about him. I know my father was honoured to have tried to work with him. These types of relationships, built on such solidarity and shared purpose, offer inspiration and hope.

The political backdrop to Eyad's time in London was uncertain and violent. The Irish Republican Army (IRA) also carried out many bombings across London. Arriving in London at this time was Alicia, my mother. She arrived in London, at just 21, coming from a small coastal town where I would grow up. It was the classic tale of a small-town girl who goes to the big city. She worked at Guy's Hospital as a nurse and accepted a blind date her friend set up one day, only agreeing after learning the man in question owned a Ford Capri!

My mother was not a left-wing political activist. Knowledge about Palestine was sparse, and at the time, there were only three TV channels. Nor did my father appear to be seeking a partner to smoke shisha and plot a revolution with either. However, my father was handsome, and they fell in love quickly. My mother's mother described him as looking like the much-admired Hollywood actor Gregory Peck. It's charming but also shows that Eyad 'passed' as non-Arab. This would have meant he would have been a victim of less racism and stereotyping. How people treated and saw him would nourish a belief that he could help promote Palestinians as more than just 'terrorists' through interpersonal relationships.

In 1975 the Palestinian revolution was at its Zenith. And not all Palestinian students on scholarships in Europe were completing their studies. Many were leaving to fight alongside the PLO and *fedayeen* in Lebanon. Many families thought their children were safe in Europe. However, they would tragically learn their son had been fighting and died in Lebanon.[10] Edward Said paid tribute to Hanna Mikhail, 'Abu Ommar'. He was an established Palestinian intellectual working at Harvard who left his security to fight in Lebanon. He tragically died on a boat travelling to Tripoli.

This story serves as a reminder for Palestinians in the diaspora. There is a constant tension of whether to stay in Europe, or to follow your heart and deepest desires, to return and work with your people, and in some cases fight alongside them.

Of Hanna Mikhail, Said wrote:

> Hanna Mikhail was a true intellectual. What I have said about him neither sentimentalizes nor exaggerates his qualities. He retained his original Quaker modesty and plainness. But, as an intellectual should, he lived according to his ideas and never tailored his democratic, secular values to suit new masters and occasions. For all Palestinians today, and in stark contrast to the great sell-out and abject surrender of our leaders, he represents a distinguished role model, a man who did not debase himself or his people. Why? Because he lived his ideas, and died for them. It is as simple as that. By his example, Hanna Mikhail admonishes those who have outlived him for a while.[11]

Peace Talks

In the context of vicious fighting and the Israeli occupation, different Palestinian factions continued to carry out missions to garner public attention. For example, the PFLP hijacked an Air France flight leaving Tel Aviv carrying 246 passengers. The passengers were mostly Jewish and Israeli. The plane ended up in Entebbe, Uganda, which led to a dramatic, and since dramatized, rescue of the passengers by Israeli commandos. The event gained global coverage but did little else politically. My father recalls everyone talking about it in London, and he felt that Palestinians were only being known for one thing: plane hijackings and violence. It was clear to him that this kind of global attention was not sufficient alone. The burgeoning peace process offered a path out of what at that time seemed like endless violence.

With his relationship blossoming, my father continued his studies but struggled with some of the exams. In addition to studying, he also worked at Barnet Hospital, coincidentally somewhere I later worked also. He told me he didn't enjoy the work. It was unfulfilling for him to prescribe medication, although he enjoyed some of the intellectual discussions concerning mental illness. In 1977 Eyad was still seeing out the final year of his Diploma in Psychiatric Medicine, but major political shifts were taking place.

The first was the arrival of Jimmy Carter as the new US president, a Democrat who signalled his support for a Palestinian state. This was a hopeful moment for Palestinians. However, the PLO would have to meet UN resolutions 242 and 338. This implied acceptance of Israel as a state. Carter gave a speech in March 1977 that indicated that Israel needed to establish permanent borders and that a homeland needed to be provided for Palestinian refugees. His comments were met with hope by some Palestinians and fear amongst some Israelis.[12] Later Carter explained his aims:

> Since I had made our nation's commitment to human rights a central tenet of our foreign policy, it was impossible for me to ignore the very serious problems on the West Bank. The continued deprivation of Palestinian rights was not only used as the primary lever against Israel, but was contrary to the basic moral and ethical principles of both our countries. In my opinion it was imperative that the United States work to obtain for these people the right to vote, the right to assemble and to debate issues that affected their lives, the right to own property without fear of its being confiscated, and the right to be free of military rule. To deny these rights was an indefensible position for a free and democratic society.[13]

The other significant change in 1977 was a stunning peace agreement between Israel and Egypt. The Egyptian President Anwar Sadat and Menachem Begin (former leader of the Irgun) had negotiated a 'land for peace' deal. Egypt was to get back the ground it lost to Israel in 1967, except for Gaza, which would remain under Israeli occupation. The deal was a significant blow to Arafat and the PLO.

In 1978 the PLO's representative Hammami, who had been signalling the PLO's desire for a 'two-state solution, was killed by Abu Nidal. Abu Nidal objected to a peace process, fearing it would only harm Palestinians' quest for justice. This was the rationale for a series of murders that started with Hammami and ended with the attempted murder of the Israeli ambassador to London.[14] The level of violence and killing in the 1970s and 1980s was astonishing. It's hard to imagine what would happen today if we saw such violence. But it serves as a reminder that many battles that only play out today in the Op-Ed pages were once far bloodier.

The media readily used Palestinian factional violence to present Palestinians as violent terrorists. However, there was still plenty of grassroots organising going on. The famous actress Vanessa Redgrave had pushed the British actors' union to boycott Israel. And she also starred in a 66-minute TV documentary about the suffering of Palestinians. A Los Angeles cinema showing the documentary was bombed. No injuries were reported, and the *New York Times* denied that the suspect had links to any militant Jewish organisation.[15] But the two events highlight the early Boycott Divestment, Sanctions (BDS) activism that was taking shape, the media's role in shaping the discussion on Israel/Palestine and the terrible state of violence taking place in the name of Palestinians and Israelis.

The life of a Palestinian in the West was something Edward Said noted in his famous book, *Orientalism*:

> The life of an Arab Palestinian in the West, particularly in America, is disheartening. There exists here an almost unanimous consensus that politically he does not exist, and when it is allowed that he does, it is either as a nuisance or as an oriental. The web of racism, cultural stereotypes, political imperialism, dehumanising ideology holding the Arab or the Muslim is very strong indeed, and it is this web which every Palestinian has come to feel as his uniquely punishing destiny.[16]

My father's time in London was the first opportunity he had to see how Palestinians were seen by the West, from the vantage of the West. He found it shocking how people would often be surprised to meet a 'well-spoken and intelligent' Palestinian. For Eyad, Palestinians were being presented as not much more than terrorists. Eyad also saw first-hand, in the pre-internet age, how the reality of life in Palestine was not reported. He understood the power of the media in shaping narratives, and he was also able to understand the power he would have as an advocate for Palestinians. He was charming, confident, and at an interpersonal level, he knew he could change minds; he just needed the opportunity.

Eyad once told me a story in which he had tried to pick a flower in Hyde Park, London. Only to be chastised by a park officer. It was this moment that he held as an example of how regimented and controlling British life was. For him, the beauty of life was somehow lost in some of its seemingly cruel methods of control and uniformity. He had found the education system a series of hoop-jumping exercises and the clinical work of psychiatry unfulfilling. He wasn't contemptuous of British life; there were many aspects he admired. However, his heart, his soul, was in Gaza, Palestine, a place where he could be himself and feel freer despite everything.

Notes

1. Al Jazeera 2009, 'PLO, History of a Revolution: Intifada', <https://www.aljazeera.com/program/plo-history-of-a-revolution/2009/8/16/plo-history-of-a-revolution-intifada>
2. "Joseph Sieff." Wikipedia, Wikimedia Foundation, <https://en.wikipedia.org/wiki/Joseph_Sieff>20th August 2020
3. Birmingham Daily Post 1974, p.1, January 2nd, retrieved from British Newspaper Archive.
4. Ibid
5. Khalidi, R 2020, *The Hundred Years' War on Palestine: A History of Settler Colonialism and Resistance, 1917–2017*, Metropolitan Books, New York, pp125
6. Al Jazeera 2020, 'Ghassan Kanafani and the era of revolutionary Palestinian media'. <https://www.aljazeera.com/program/the-listening-post/2020/7/19/ghassan-kanafani-and-the-era-of-revolutionary-palestinian-media>
7. Ibid
8. Avnery, U 1986, *My Friend the Enemy*, Zed Books, London, pp35
9. Ibid
10. Abu Sitta, S 2016, *Mapping My Return: A Palestinian Memoir*, The American University in Cairo Press, Cairo, pp243
11. Said E, 'A Tribute to Abu Omar', retrieved on August 23rd 2021 <https://www.abu-omar-hanna.info/spip/spip.php?article103>
12. Alam, M 1992, 'Carter, Camp David and the Issue of Palestine', *Pakistan Horizon* Vol. 45, No. 1 (January), pp. 75-83
13. Thrall, N 2017, *The Only Language They Understand: Forcing Compromise in Israel and Palestine*, Metropolitan Books, New York, pp14

14. Hitchens, C 2002, 'The terrorist I knew', *The Guardian*, August 25th
15. Harmetz, A 1978, 'Theater for Redgrave Film Bombed', *New York Times*, June 16th
16. Said, E 1978, *Orientalism*, Pantheon Books, New York, pp27

7. THE CLINICIAN AND THE ACTIVIST

> *I started as a physician in Gaza and did not want to be involved in politics. But many of my patients were victims of torture and I became drawn into advocacy. Defending human rights is my major obsession.*
>
> —Eyad Sarraj

Eyad, now 'Dr Eyad', was returning to his beloved Gaza. His life so far had been a heavy mix of political activism, world-class mental health training and eschewing tribalism in favour of independence and critical thinking. These themes were to become his guiding forces. Dr Eyad was now Gaza's first trained psychiatrist, an extraordinary achievement and milestone. In a BBC 'Hard Talk with Tim Sebastian' interview in 1997, Eyad describes why he returned to Gaza:

> I love my people, I love my home, and I feel a kind of responsibility to help people here. What am I if I live in England and practice psychiatry? There are 5,000, 10,000 psychiatrists there. Here I can help not just my own people, it is humanity that needs help, this is what brought me back, and this is what will keep me here.[1]

As the only psychiatrist with such status and privileged knowledge, it represented an opportunity to pioneer mental health treatment. However, things would not be easy at first. Many resented the arrival of Eyad to Gaza's quaint health system. With his new foreign credentials, locals considered him flashy. Preferring their own fiefdoms, they initially stymied his attempts to start a mental health treatment unit.[2] The need for a mental health unit was critical. Once, there was no treatment if you were experiencing severe distress such as psychosis, clinical depression, schizophrenia. Eyad's idea was to replicate the model he had seen operational in London and establish Gaza's first ward. This ward would be 10-16 beds with an attending psychiatrist and nurses. In simple terms, patients would be treated on the ward before being discharged back into the community.

The Palestinian Director at Shifa Hospital opposed the move on baseless grounds. Undeterred and realising what had worked for him in the past when his good ideas were not taken up, Eyad took the radical option of approaching the WHO and Israel. But, of course, as Gaza was under occupation, real power lay with Israel and the international agencies. In approaching Israel, Eyad would encounter Israel's right-wing party members: Likud. Members of this party were known as 'Likudniks' and were often Jews from Europe who emigrated to Israel in 1948. In addition, Moshe Arens, a member of Israel's parliament, and a future minister was in contact with Eyad over health administration issues.

On meeting Moshe, Eyad said:

> I met him because I wanted to establish a clinic in Gaza. Other Palestinian doctors were opposing me. I explained my story to him, but I didn't complain about people who weren't there. He said, 'Are you sure you're an Arab? Everyone comes here to complain about the others behind their backs.' I said that I just wanted to finish this business by dealing with it. He said, 'I like this attitude,' and we became friends.[3]

After this meeting, a WHO delegation then visited Gaza, and an Israeli, Dr Lasch, took the situation seriously enough to grant the request. As a result, a small 16-bed unit was established in an eye hospital. Appalling for a population of one million. Under-resourced mental health treatment in Gaza in 1978 is not surprising: in London, in 2021, there are often mental health bed shortages. Nevertheless, this was a small victory, and Eyad could at least begin to transfer his privileged knowledge.

Being Gaza's only psychiatrist, Eyad's services were in demand. In an interview, Eyad recalls an event concerning an outbreak of fainting among schoolgirls who lived near settlements:

> It started in the West Bank,' Eyad said. 'The news spread that settlers were poisoning the schools with gas. I was appointed head of a medical committee, and I examined the cases myself. My decision was that the girls should be turned away from hospitals and sent back home. A doctor said, 'You can't do that. The PLO will shoot you!' I said, 'I'm a doctor, not a politician.[4]

Eyad's intervention was so helpful that Arens appointed him to investigate all medical negligence. If it was for the rights and health of Palestinians, Eyad was willing to work with Israelis. This decision can be seen as capitulation from the outside looking in. However, Palestinians in occupied Palestine are faced with complex moral dilemmas. Boycotting Israel – for Palestinians – is not always the best option. In this regard, Eyad was not ideologically pure or dogmatic. Nor was he trying to play to a base of BDS supporters. On the contrary, his principles of intellectual honesty and his commitment to reducing suffering were his guiding forces.

Alongside his public work, Eyad was also trying to establish extra income. He decided to do this through private clinic work. My mother, a nurse, was working alongside him. She recalls how the set-up in the home was possibly contributing to patients' treatment outcomes:

> There was this charming psychiatrist, the first of his kind, and me, an English nurse, who was administering neurological tests... it was the equivalent of going to Harley Street in London.

According to my mother, Eyad was having such great success with medication, and treatment protocols, that he was considered a 'witch doctor'. She recalls a great clamour amongst those who could afford it to be seen by Eyad.

Amongst the Gazan elites and middle classes, he was single-handedly shifting attitudes about mental illness. At that time, mental illness in Gaza was seen or explained as a curse. Evil eye, magic (voodoo), *jinn* were all beliefs rooted in pre-Islamic traditions/folk beliefs.[5] Religious and traditional healers hold much sway in communities like Gaza, and they can often use their authority and charisma to manipulate patients. Stigma, more broadly, can have many negative impacts not limited to access to treatment. For example, just seeing a psychiatrist can end a marriage in some parts of Palestine. Any hint of 'mental illness' could undermine the chance of finding a partner.

The professionalisation of mental health permitted new narratives about mental illness. One paradoxical consequence of the occupation is that clinicians have been able to situate mental health as a reaction to the occupation. This is something Eyad developed as a theory. He helped patients see their reactions to stress and violence as normal. Eyad explained that many mental health symptoms are connected to the struggle for a national cause. In some sense, these are battle scars rather than signs of weakness, and therefore worthy of respect.[6]

The arrival to Gaza of a professional mental health discourse was significant. It acted as a cultural buffer against potentially more harmful treatments and illness narratives. Eyad was at the forefront of this revolution and was developing a reputation as an authority on mental health and a man of purpose, willing to do controversial things to improve Palestinian life.

Violent Divisions

In the context of the Palestinian struggle for freedom, fraternal violence continued. Abu Nidal was killing PLO representatives active in or supportive of peace negotiations. Sadat, seeking peace with Israel, remained unpopular and was a target for those that opposed his ideas. Even close family members to Eyad were involved in amateurish plans to kill Sadat. One family member tried to smuggle dynamite into Cairo. They were arrested and had to be smuggled out through bribes. The story serves as a dramatic reminder that family kinship doesn't protect against violence as a means. Moreover, Palestinians were divided factionally and within families. This was a division that had been sowed and fuelled by Israel. And from the 1970s onwards, more division would continue to rip families apart and harm efforts toward Palestinian unity.

As Jimmy Carter pursued peace, the Palestinians were somewhat united behind the PLO. The West Bank and Gaza were seen as one political bloc. And as one political entity, there was the possibility of one Palestinian state. In this setting, the US was now engaged in serious and expansive talks with the PLO – much to the ire of Israel.[7] Eyad, like other Palestinians, was hopeful that things were changing for the better. However, a setback was suffered when the Israeli Likud party (Likudniks) was elected.

The Likud party contained members like Ariel Sharon who wanted to increase settlements in the Occupied Territories, including Gaza. This idea ran contrary to a crucial part of peace talks: returning land to Palestinians. Likud's leader was Menachem Begin, from Poland, whose parents and brother had been executed. Begin viewed the world as dangerous and antisemitic.[8] These were the types of people now in charge of Israel. Their early experiences shaped their view of the world and marked the start of what is often described as Israel's 'shift to the right'. A shift that severely hindered chances of compromise.

In 1978, at Camp David, where US presidents often conduct such meetings, Carter hosted Sadat and Begin. The talks did not go well: neither party was willing to concede. Eventually, the deadlock was broken by way of Israel, suggesting that Palestinians could govern themselves – temporarily – while a more comprehensive solution was found. Meanwhile, the Sinai would be returned to Egypt. A win for Egypt; the Palestinians, however, were left empty-handed and felt forgotten. Tragically, this 'temporary' solution of an autonomous Palestinian government still exists today. This lack of progress for Palestinians didn't deter Egypt from striking a peace deal with Israel in 1978.

In 1982 Israel invaded Lebanon. The attack was led by the defence minister and future Israeli Prime Minister, Ariel Sharon. This operation was aimed at destroying the PLO. During their time in Lebanon, the PLO had become stronger, and Israel saw the opportunity to end Palestinian statehood aspirations.[9] It was a brutal campaign, and more than 19,000 Palestinians and Lebanese, mostly civilians, were killed and more than 30,000 wounded. It also led to massacres in two refugee camps: Sabra and Shatila. Israel's overwhelming use of force from the air had all the hallmarks of their approach to Gaza: the complete disregard for the loss of civilian life and the sowing of widespread fear. The historian Rashid Khalidi cites a letter Begin sent to Reagan during this time:

> In an August 5th letter to Ronald Reagan, Begin wrote that 'these days' he felt as if he and his 'valiant army' were 'facing 'Berlin' where, amongst

innocent civilians, Hitler and his henchmen hide in a bunker deep beneath the surface.[10]

The insight into the mind of Begin offers some clues about the paranoia, fear, and violence of which Eyad was to become aware. Eyad considered the possibility that the traumas the Jewish community experienced in Europe would somehow manifest against Palestinians. This underlying belief often guided his approach to peace that violent resistance would only trigger something deeper and more destructive from within the collective Jewish psyche.[11] He also felt that violence would concede Palestinians' moral high ground.

In August 1982, after ten weeks of fighting, the PLO left Lebanon. With the PLO in exile, Gaza remained under Israeli occupation. The demise of the PLO had left a political vacuum, and the growing movement in Gaza towards Islamic politics was primed to fill it. Many assume Gaza to have always been conservative. However, Gaza for many decades was a much more liberal society. In Gaza, my mother recalls smoking shisha, swimming in the sea and wearing short skirts. Of course, it wasn't like Western Europe, but the prevalence of Islamic influenced social norms was far less than we see today in Gaza.

In theory, the rise of political Islamism in Gaza during this period, exacerbated by Israeli policies, pitted Islamists against Nationalists.[12] This led to increased tension and fighting between Fatah and members of the Muslim Brotherhood (the precursor to Hamas) and increased resistance against Israeli's occupying forces. Tensions, and acts of resistance, were only exacerbated when Israel announced it would increase settlement construction in Gaza. With the situation deteriorating, the PLO in exile, and peace talks looking hopeless, things in Palestine were reaching boiling point.

Shifa Hospital

One of Eyad's dearest friends was an academic working at Harvard, Sara Roy. Sara, an author of many books and essays about Gaza, is often referred to as a leading authority on Gaza.[13] Sara coined the term 'de-development'. It was a theoretical frame to explain how Israel systematically undermines any chance of Gaza developing an economy.[14] Aside from her vast knowledge, one of the other reasons she is so credible on Gaza is that, since 1985, she has been visiting regularly and maintaining relationships with people in Gaza.

Sara first met Eyad at Marna House Hotel, a hotel that still exists today. It remains a historic meeting place for many visitors to Gaza.

On first meeting Eyad, she recalls his 'fierce honesty, and absence of any sense of caution or tentativeness...he was open, direct and resolute'.[15] In 1986, when

Sara re-returned to Gaza to document health conditions, the Israeli military government denied her entry to Shifa hospital. Sara writes:

> When Eyad showed up at Marna House, he greeted me warmly, and we had the following exchange:
> 'Let's go, Sara.'
> 'Let's go where,' I asked?
> 'Shifa.'
> 'Shifa? You mean you got me permission?'
> 'No, you will never get permission, and when you are inside the hospital, you will understand why. I shall bring you in because you must see for yourself the conditions in the hospital.'
> 'Eyad, you could get into serious trouble with the authorities. You might lose your job. I don't want you to take such risks for me, and I am not asking you to.'
> 'I am not worried. But you must write about what you see, about everything I show you.'

At considerable risk to himself—and it was only later that I learned from others how great the risk actually was—Eyad surreptitiously brought me into Shifa, walking me through the entire hospital including the operating room. He allowed me to take as much time as I needed despite the worried looks of the hospital staff. He did not say too much, but he did not have to; conditions inside the hospital were appalling as the following excerpt from my published report, *The Gaza Strip Survey*, shows:

> 'Mice, roaches and other insects were observed scurrying through individual wards, rooms and bathrooms. Rooms were extremely dirty and in a state of decay as indicated by broken windows, peeling paint and cracked floors. Hospital beds were old and rusting and patients were observed two to a bed, lying on sheets that were torn and blood-stained. Hospital personnel indicated that the same sheets are often used for more than one patient due to a lack of supplies. Rooms are cleaned only when patients can afford to pay... The surgical operating room [was] in a similar state of deterioration and extremely unsterile; cigarette butts were observed on the floor of the [OR].

This one paragraph caught the attention of the international media, and a firestorm ensued, including a four-minute segment on life inside Gaza on the ABC evening news. Eyad told me that the Palestinian director of the hospital was fired and that hospital conditions soon improved but only temporarily. After Shifa was cleaned up and repaired, the military government invited various international groups and organisations into the hospital as a way of refuting my claims.

The Knesset even threatened to subpoena Meron and me since they accused us of having been paid by the PLO to write the report![16]

The story encapsulates the types of struggles Eyad was facing. As a trusted and reliable communicator, foreign visitors would visit Eyad for advice and information. These relationships were opportunities to get messages out to a Western audience, and Eyad understood the power of the media in shaping public opinion. In addition, he was learning how to use his skills, experience and growing confidence to score small but important victories against the Israeli apparatus.

Intifada (انتفاضة) / Uprising

> *Suicide bombers of today were the children of the first Intifada. The 'children of the stone' were not made of stone* – Eyad Sarraj

Family life in Gaza was not my mother's first choice. As a young woman from Hampshire, she understandably struggled with life in Gaza. Due to unsanitary conditions, she faced numerous illnesses and viral diseases. And despite learning Arabic, loving Eyad and making friends with other expatriates in Gaza, she never quite settled. They tried to settle in Cornwall in 1986, and for a while, we all lived as a family. I vaguely recall being on my father's shoulders picking apples from a tree, feeding cows at the bottom of the garden, and going on family outings. My father tried to enjoy his work at a local psychiatric hospital but found the large bureaucratic NHS stifling and the patients' Cornish accents hard to discern. So despite renaming our family house Falastin (Palestine) and having relatives living nearby, Gaza was always on his mind.

The *Intifada*, 'uprising' in Arabic, was pivotal in Palestinian history. After an Israeli car crashed into Gaza workers, a wave of non-violent protests erupted across Palestine. They included strikes and boycotts. Israel reacted with an 'Iron Fist' policy—and the policy was to 'break bones' and 'skulls' of protestors.[17] Young people suffered greatly, and between 1988 – 1990 up to 30,000 children received beatings that required medical attention. One third were under the age of ten.[18] These images were being shown worldwide, and Israel's image was being tarnished. For the first time, Israel was seen as a brutal occupying power. The infamous photos of kids with stones against tanks became etched into popular conscience.

THE CLINICIAN AND THE ACTIVIST | 55

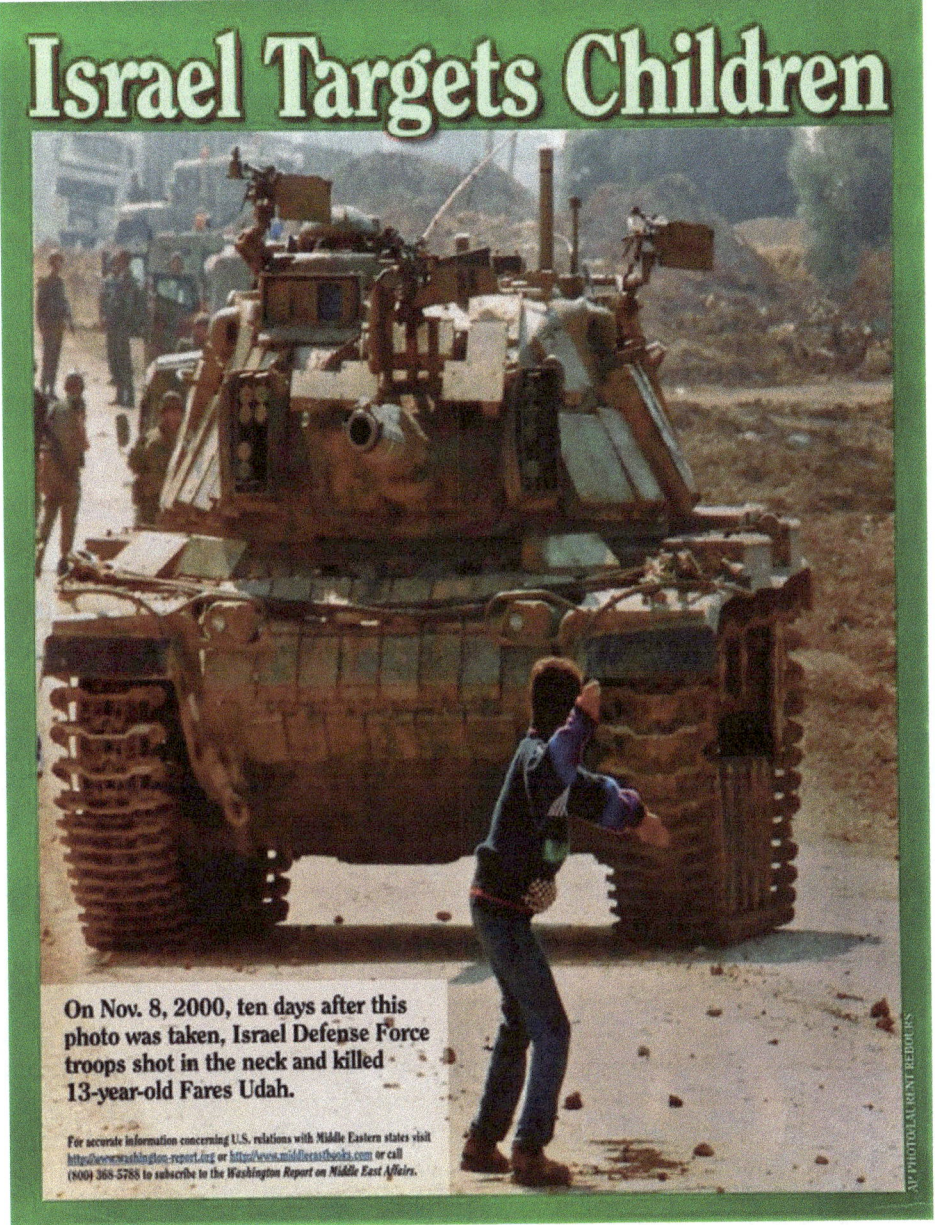

A colour poster showing Fares throwing stones on an Israeli tank in Gaza in 2000. www.palarchive.org

Eyad could not stay in England anymore, and the violence in Gaza meant that it was not a place for his young family. So his return to Gaza was inevitable.

Back to Work

In Gaza, Eyad immediately responded to the violence. He took up extra shifts at Shifa hospital and helped treat the wounded.[19] Eyad was acutely aware that an entire generation was now being exposed to trauma. He worried about the psychological wounds that this generation would have to carry. He also felt the violence that Israel enacted would only serve to move their society further down the path of normalising more brutal forms of violence.

Eyad also continued to play host to visiting delegations. On this occasion, he was hosting a group of Israeli physicians. These were brave Israelis who wanted to see the impact of Israel's policies for themselves. One of the group's members was to become a long-time friend of Eyad's, Ruchama Marton. Ruchama was also a psychiatrist and psychotherapist and had served, like almost all Israelis, in the Israeli army.

Eyad spoke at length with the delegation and put them at ease in his own way. He was encouraging and emphasised the importance of witnessing what was happening in Gaza. These sets of relationships that Eyad was nurturing helped lay the groundwork for Palestinian–Israeli Physicians for Human Rights (PIPHR). Founded in 1988, PIPHR would advocate for 'a just society where the right to health is granted equally to all people under Israel's responsibility.'[20] It's an organisation that still exists today and has tremendous moral authority.

Using the power of their relationship to espouse universal humanism, Eyad & Ruchama would travel the world speaking at conferences. It was also a worldview that did not shy away from speaking honestly about the oppression they witnessed. During one conference in Canada, Ruchama was accused of being a traitor, which I am sure was also levelled at Eyad. Ruchama, with great passion, responded thus:

> In 1956, when Eyad, then a twelve-year-old boy, was being forced into a cellar with an Israeli gun at his back, she was a nineteen-year-old Israel Defense Forces (IDF) conscript stationed with the Givati Brigade in the Sinai desert. A group of thirty or so surrendering Egyptian soldiers approached their position. Exhausted, thirsty, and hungry, they begged for food and water. An Israeli officer ordered their execution; the men were shot. The massacre changed her forever. She had seen what 'purity of arms' meant in action, and never again could turn a blind eye to crimes of the state or to the complicity of her fellow citizens. 'That's why I am here tonight with Eyad,' she said. 'Maybe I don't live at peace with my society, but I can almost be at peace with myself.'[21]

Eyad and Ruchama were caught in their people's traumatic histories. They both had the option of repressing their memories and living a life of comfort. Instead, they chose to use their unique positions in society to benefit all. In doing so, they would be living a life of purpose, but not without cost to themselves. Their cooperation had got Eyad into trouble, and Israel refused to let him back. He found himself effectively deported by Israeli authorities, ending any hopes of cross border work.

In an interview with the Canadian magazine Equinox, Eyad recounted his interaction with an Israeli soldier during the First Intifada:

> He [Eyad] was once stopped during the Intifada and ordered by an Israeli soldier to extinguish flames from a burning tire with his bare hands. He refused the order. When the soldier threatened to take his identification card, el-Sarraj didn't protest. 'Go ahead, take it, I don't care,' he said. And when the soldier threatened to beat him, el-Sarraj said, 'Go ahead, but before you do, I know there is a real human being behind that uniform, and I would like you to show me that person.' The soldier got tears in his eyes, and then he just walked away.[22]

Out of Place

Reeling from political events, Eyad would benefit from some time away from Gaza. He was very fortunate to be allowed to take a sabbatical at Oxford University. He had been invited to Oxford by refugee scholar Barbara Harrell-Bond and would be a resident at the Refugee Studies Centre. He spent the year in the company of academics and intellectuals and giving talks. He once remarked that he wished he had used the opportunity differently. He wasn't a natural scholar, but he absorbed other people's ideas and reflected on the different ways people saw the world. In his own way, he was an intellectual.

I recall visiting Oxford to see my father. This was my first taste of a world of intellectuals and academics. We went to an enormous townhouse in Oxford. There were lots of – to me – unfamiliar objects, like African art, handmade Arabic rugs, sculptures, black and white photographs, original looking maps, and piles of books everywhere. We ate French cheese and bread, and the adults drank red wine. I was from a small English town, and this was my first taste of what I now know as a well-off, left-wing academic culture.

This group probably comprises quite a significant section of Palestinian support worldwide. These people use their institutions, connections, intellect, and moral courage to help Palestinians. But they were worlds away from my childhood – and from my father's in many ways. Yet, while alien to this world, Eyad was also more comfortable than other Palestinians. He was quick to adapt, and his intellectual curiosity helped him fit in.

An obvious parallel is the cosmopolitan and intellectual Edward Said. Said, in his memoir, described his experiences of never truly fitting in. Eyad empathised and remarked once that people in Gaza thought he was 'schizophrenic'.[23] They felt he was trying to be European because of his habits and ideals. He was indeed out of place – both in Gaza and abroad – but he loved Gaza, he was Palestinian, and all he wanted was to improve life for himself and his community.

Between 1988 and the early 1990s, there had been a series of political events that would foreshadow the infamous Oslo Peace Process. In 1988 Jordan gave up its claim to the West Bank, and with the West Bank back in the Palestinian orbit, Arafat would declare a Palestinian state. Arafat's declaration was very rhetorical, but it meant that Palestinians were publicly seeking to control their destiny. Arafat and the PLO were putting all their eggs in the basket of US-backed peace talks.

To garner further US support Arafat publicly announced an end to all forms of terrorism. Given the US's significant funding to Israel, they were viewed as the only global power that could help nurture an agreement between Palestinians and Israel.[24] However, other Palestinian factions were sceptical of such a concession. This strategic difference led to further violence. For example, the PLFP launched an attack on an Israeli beach. The aim, which was later revealed, was to undermine peace talks between Arafat and the US.[25] However, despite Arafat's best efforts to win over the US, the peace talks went nowhere. Arafat was left a demoralised figure in a political landscape that showed little sign of hope.

Notes

1. BBC 1997, *Hard Talk*, 'Tim Sebastian interviews Dr Eyad Sarraj'
2. Aaron, P 2016, 'The Pathological Optimist: One Man's Vision for Palestinian Well-Being', *Journal of Palestine Studies*, V45(2)
3. Neslen, A 2011, *In Your Eyes a Sandstorm. Ways of Being Palestinian*, University of California Press, US, pp256
4. Neslen, A 2011, *In Your Eyes a Sandstorm. Ways of Being Palestinian*, University of California Press, US, pp257
5. Limm, A 2018, 'The Attribution of Mental Health Problems to Jinn: An Explorative Study in a Transcultural Psychiatric Outpatient Clinic', *Front Psychiatry*, 9 (89)
6. Mahmoud Daher, interview with Tom Hill, 2015
7. Khalidi, R 2020, *The Hundred Years' War on Palestine: A History of Settler Colonialism and Resistance, 1917–2017*, Metropolitan Books, New York, pp135

8. Thrall, N 2017, *The Only Language They Understand: Forcing Compromise in Israel and Palestine*, Metropolitan Books, New York, pp16

9. Al Jazeera 2009, 'PLO, History of a Revolution: Intifada', <https://www.aljazeera.com/program/plo-history-of-a-revolution/2009/8/16/plo-history-of-a-revolution-intifada>

10. Khalidi, R 2020, *The Hundred Years' War on Palestine: A History of Settler Colonialism and Resistance, 1917–2017*, Metropolitan Books, New York, pp147

11. Kemp, M. 2011, *Thinking Space: Dehumanization, Guilt, and Large-group Dynamics with Reference to the West, Israel, and the Palestinians*, Routledge, London

12. Baroud, R 2009, *My Father Was a Freedom Fighter: Gaza's Untold Story*, Pluto Press, London, pp138

13. Roy, S, Bio, *Harvard* website <https://cmes.fas.harvard.edu/people/sara-roy>

14. Roy, S 1995, *The Gaza Strip: The Political Economy of De-Development*, Institute for Palestine Studies, US

15. Roy, S 2015, Sara Roy Tribute to Eyad, *Gaza Mental Health Foundation*, <https://www.gazamentalhealth.org/wp-content/uploads/2015/04/sara_roy_Tribute_to_Eyad.pdf>

16. Ibid

17. Dacey, R. 1998, 'Risk attitude, punishment, and the Intifada'. *Conflict Management and Peace Science*, Vol. 16, No. 1, Spring, 1998, pp. 77-88

18. Aaron, P 2016, 'The Pathological Optimist: One Man's Vision for Palestinian Well-Being', *Journal of Palestine Studies*, V45(2)

19. Ibid

20. Physicians for Human Rights, 'About Us' <https://www.phr.org.il/en/>

21. Aaron, P 2016, 'The Pathological Optimist: One Man's Vision for Palestinian Well-Being', *Journal of Palestine Studies*, V45(2)

22. Said, E, 2000, *Out of Place: A Memoir*, Penguin House, New York

23. National Public Radio (NPR) 2001, 'Fresh Air Archive: Interviews with Terry Gross. July 30th 2001. Eyad El-Sarraj'. [online] Available at: <https://freshairarchive.org/segments/eyad-el-sarraj> [Accessed 1 October 2021].

24. Ruebner, J, 'Bringing Assistance to Israel in Line With Rights and U.S. Laws', *Carnegie Endowment International*, May 12th, 2001. <https://carnegieendowment.org/2021/05/12/bringing-assistance-to-israel-in-line-with-rights-and-u.s.-laws-pub-84503>

25. Al Jazeera 2009, 'PLO, History of a Revolution: Intifada', <https://www.aljazeera.com/program/plo-history-of-a-revolution/2009/8/16/plo-history-of-a-revolution-intifada>

8. THE GAZA COMMUNITY MENTAL HEALTHCARE PROGRAMME

In 1990 Eyad returned to Gaza from Oxford. He had worked primarily in large health institutions, such as acute mental health hospitals, up to this point. These experiences offered limited fulfilment, and he yearned for something that would allow him to treat mental health as both an environmental and an individual issue. His European colleagues would help steer him towards this goal.

Over the years, Eyad visited Europe and the US, lecturing and connecting with European physicians and academics. Two such academics who would feature in Eyad's life were David Henley and Henrik Pelling. Eyad met them in Stockholm, Sweden, in May 1988, where he spoke at an event sponsored by the Swedish Palestine Solidarity Association entitled: 'Israel-40 Years-Myth and Reality'. After the event, Eyad spent time in Uppsala meeting up with David and Henrik. They write:

> Eyad had some general ideas concerning starting a Mental Health Center but the specifics were unclear. He was concerned with vulnerable groups in society, particularly children. Instead of giving them guidance and protection from all the violence around them, myths were made that they were leading the resistance by, for example, throwing stones at Israeli tanks. Women also suffered under the conservative social mores as well as the ongoing destruction of the family. Many men who had also spent long periods of time in Israeli prisons under severe conditions also needed help when released.
>
> Eyad was also worried about the stigma associated with mental health care. In addition to a very strong general aversion to visiting a clinic associated with mental health, the only exposure people in Gaza had had was that of a 'last resort', mental health hospital. How could one begin to break down this stigma? And then there was no infrastructure, finances, or professional personnel, and not even an interest in mental health. One would have to begin from the beginning. Eyad has subsequently written, or voiced the opinion, that it was in Uppsala, Sweden that he had started to formulate his plans for GCMHP.[1]

With a rough plan sketched out, Eyad returned to Gaza in 1990, and not long later, the Gaza Community Mental Health Program (GCMHP) was established. He was initially lent a home (to use as an office/clinic) by a relative. However, after drawing upon support from the local community and using his political connections, he secured his first $100,000 grant. Eyad's charisma, credentials, competence, and political independence helped.

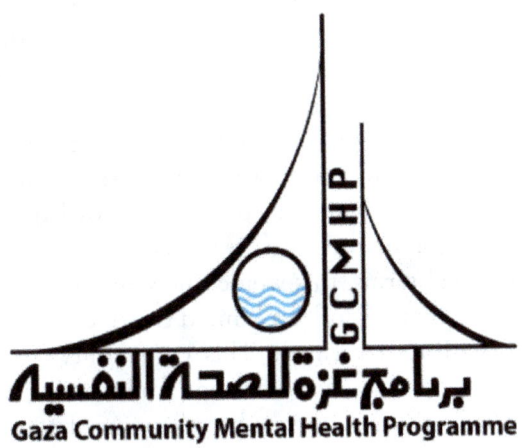

Gaza Community Mental Health Programme

Meanwhile, in Hampshire, where my mother, myself, and brother lived, we were tasked with designing a logo for GCMHP. My brother used a newly purchased Apple Mac to use a rudimentary design program to create GCMHP's logo. The only creative direction was that Eyad wanted it to be inspired by the sea. The logo my brother eventually designed is the same one used today.

GCMHP, the first centre of its kind, had an enormous challenge ahead. It would be tasked with breaking down negative attitudes to mental illness, introducing new language and new ideas about mental health, using both nuanced cultural and western knowledge to treat victims of political violence, training a professional workforce, and striving to link mental health to human rights. All of this would be done in the context of Israel's occupation. An occupying force that not only controlled the movement of Palestinians but also engaged in collective punishments: home demolition, imprisonment, house raids, and iterations of physical violence.

In its first six-seven years, GCMHP grew rapidly. One of the external reasons for this growth was the significant uptick in donor aid channelled through the Occupied Palestinian Territories (OPT). Following a World Bank plan called 'Investment in Peace', around $23 Billion of development money has since been spent in the OPT.[2] The aim was to support a new Palestinian state-building program. However, many observers have concluded that this money has not improved Palestinians' lives sustainably. It has also let Israel off the hook for its responsibilities and provided cover for Israel to continue violently dispossessing Palestinians of their land.[3]

By 1997 GCMHP had three outreach clinics based in refugee camps and boasted 70 staff, eleven clinicians working with children and their families (one psychiatrist, six psychologists, one general practitioner, one nurse and two social workers). About 1200 new service users were being referred annually. 45% of these were children, 72% were refugees, and the male to female ratio was 55:45. Most families self-referred into the service, and a range of treatments was offered.[4] They had also pioneered a hotline that allowed potential patients to receive support over the telephone.

One of the significant problems GCMHP faced, especially when trying to scale a service to help a large community, was the limited number of trained staff. To overcome this, GCMHP attempted to transfer knowledge from those already trained back into the community, e.g., teachers, school counsellors, and recreational staff. In practical terms, this would allow teachers to detect behavioural problems in schools, potentially offer a limited treatment, and in most cases refer pupils back to GCMHP for treatment. This 'community' approach was the cornerstone of GCMHP's work. It was different from the WHO's more prevalent mode: a model in which the doctor was the sole point of contact, often only prescribing psychiatric medication.

The second strand to building a workforce was creating GCMHP's own Post Graduate Diploma. In an exciting cooperation with seven universities around the world, a curriculum was developed that fused scientific evidence with practical local experience. The result provided Gaza with a regular supply of mental health practitioners. Modules from the community diploma continue to include: stress and trauma, ethics, child psychopathology, and statistics. And even when COVID-19 reached Gaza, GCMHP switched to distance learning with students being taught via Zoom. GCMHP, operating within a public health model, also trained psychiatry students and nurses from local universities. Cohorts would be taught theoretical and practical training, focusing on clinical interviews, diagnosis of mental disorders and therapy management plans. The overall impact of these training and institutional connections gave rise to a new mental health discourse in Gaza and more effective treatment for those in distress.

In the early '90s, Eyad's open borders, open minds approach led him to invite Israeli psychiatrists, such as Ruchama Marton, to assist with GCMHP's work. Ruchama volunteered with other Israeli colleagues to train GCMHP's staff. Contact was even made with Tel Aviv University's Psychology Department, which started to carry out supervision and training. However, this bold initiative was terminated when Israel no longer permitted Palestinian students to come to Tel Aviv for their studies. It's hard to imagine this sort of Israeli/Palestinian cooperation happening today. For some, this might be seen as progress; for others, it may seem like an opportunity lost.

Of course, mental health workers' context in Gaza is uniquely challenging. All Palestine's inhabitants live under occupation and are deeply affected by violence, including the hard-working therapists, who themselves are trying to offer a form of stoic compassion. As one GCMHP staff member put it, Eyad tried to tend to the needs of the therapists:

> We were in it together, side by side: not him as a remote and mysterious figure. He made us feel that he needed us, that he was interested in our inner lives, in our hopes. He was our collective therapist.[5]

Surprisingly, Eyad was not that well trained in psychotherapy. The standard for the era in which he studied, his psychiatry training did not include a therapy component. Despite this, he had an intuitive understanding of people, was deeply reflective and curious, and his manner was warm and comforting. This approach has been described as 'central relatedness'.[6] He would try to see the person in front of him, the person – or soul – underneath all the layers. This was his approach to people in general, patients in particular, and Israelis. Despite this idiosyncratic approach, much evidence has pointed to the importance of the relationship in psychotherapy.[7] Eyad's genuine relationship-building abilities gave him an edge in the world of psychotherapy.

A Community in Treatment

In 2010 I taught a group of 16- or 17-year-olds at Gaza's American International School. Operation Cast Lead (the war on Gaza) in 2009-2010 was a very recent memory, and its consequences impacted many of our conversations. It soon became clear from talking to the group that over years of living in Gaza, not one of these young people did not know someone who died, had lost a loved one or witnessed violence. Eyad had keenly observed this shocking development. He reflected that he did remember a time in the community when a single death would be painfully felt. It's hard to delineate the impact of violence on individuals; we all bring something different to the experience. Our coping methods vary, and while it is a science, it remains imperfect.

In Gaza, GCMHP were at the forefront of studying the impact of violence. A core team of GCMHP staff, people like Abdel Aziz Thabet, Abdel Hamid Afana and Samir Qouta, were highly prolific, carrying out vital research published in well-known scientific journals. One GCMHP study, of a randomly selected group of 2779 children, showed that during the first *Intifada with* the following results: 95% had been tear-gassed, 52% beaten, 35% detained briefly, 11% imprisoned, 50% had had a family member detained, 97% houses raided by the army, 37% witnessed the beating of family members, 3% extended family member killed and 11% experienced house demolition.[8] Indeed, it has been reported that children were 40% more likely to die a violent death in Gaza than in the West Bank.[9]

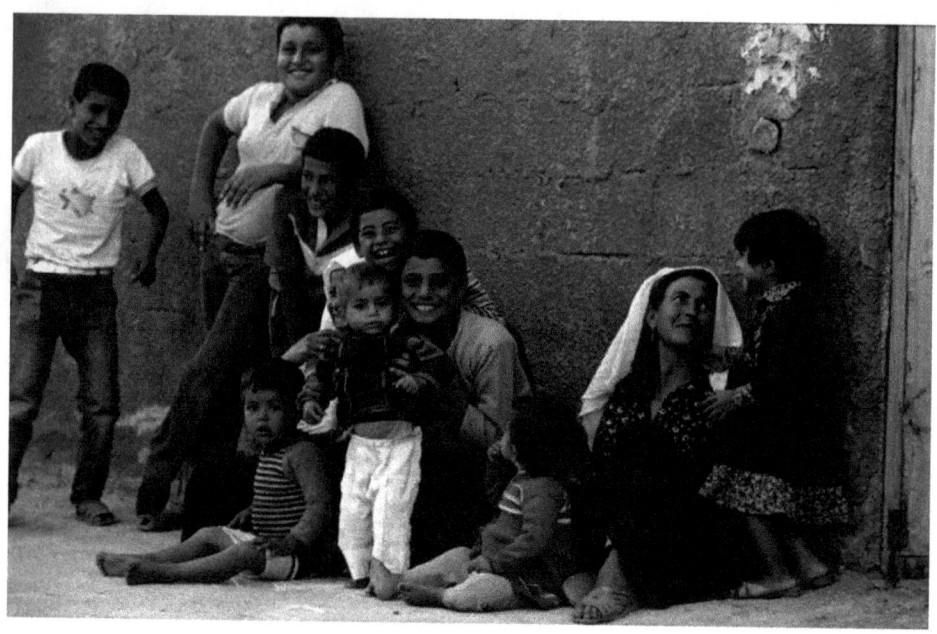

Children with their mothers sitting in a Jabalia Palestinian Refugee Camp street, north of the Gaza Strip in 1987." www.palarchive.org

In this violent context, Eyad often theorized about the father's role. He believed strongly that the father offered children a crucial symbolic and material protection source. He often overheard children ask questions like: 'How could he (the father) protect me if he could not protect himself?' Eyad believed that in the minds of many children, the father's image of protection and safety was erased and replaced with a new image of powerlessness and defeat. Eyad had observed this during play therapy in summer camps. One of the children's favourite games, Eyad says, was often called 'Arabs and Jews'. Eyad found it telling to see many of them choose to be Jews, not Arabs. He noted that for them, a Jew meant power. However, the children quickly realized that their new hero was also the enemy, so the image was rejected but left a vacuum of anxiety.

Children were anxious to find a replacement for the father figure, but they also needed a powerful figure to look up to. Eyad considered that this necessary powerful figure could take many forms: charismatic Imams, community leaders, militias, or political parties. These people and spaces offered a haven that nurtured feelings of security and protection. Eyad saw how the group(s)/individuals could become the new family that replaces the father. Considering the impact of this environment on future generations, Eyad believed that violence would breed hopelessness and motivate more extreme forms of violence. He warned:

> The stone throwing youth of the 1st Intifada are now the suicide bombers of the 2nd Intifada, and we are not sure how we will describe the next generation.[10]

In this socio-political context, GCMHP, being the first centre of its kind, had a critical and complex role in providing treatment. In an interview, Eyad described the approach he favoured with a typical case:

> **Eyad**: A typical case of today, is a case of a young boy who is around 12 and started bed-wetting very recently, although he has been, like, dry for the last nine years or so. And the bed-wetting, today, is due to the acute trauma–being subjected to some kind of severe blast of the Israeli bombs or terrible scene in TV of people being shot or killed, blood. Or being harassed here and there, or through the fear coming from the eyes of his mother or his father, who are usually terrified, and in a state of panic, unable to protect their children.
>
> Children usually ask, 'Why don't you have a gun, Father? How are you going to protect me if the Israelis are going to shoot–if the Israeli soldiers are going to do something, how are you going to protect me?' So, the father is usually helpless and the mother is in a state of panic, and then the end result is a child who is bed-wetting, sometimes unable to concentrate in the school, sometimes unable to behave well, sometimes violent.
>
> **Interviewer**: So what can you do for the 12-year-old boy who's wetting his bed?
>
> **Eyad**: Well, you see, we have different ways, and sometimes we mix them together, but the basic thing is to make the child understand why it is happening to him, and to make the family understand why is it happening to a child, and then how to cope with this. The minute you have the insight, as a child, into this problem then you actually have 50 percent chance of improvement. And the other methods we use are behavioral, kind of, conditioning. And then we also sometimes use medications, but it has to be all done in the context of the family setting, where really people understand why this is happening to them and the child should understand why it is happening to him. Without this, it can go on for a long time.[11]

While each case is different, there was an acute understanding of integrated systems of power that start with the family, broaden to society and end with the occupation. Situating the individual within these systems forced the patient and therapist to confront the role of power in all aspects of their lives.

Hasan Ziada, a clinical psychologist at GCMHP, is acutely aware of the impact of demoralization, violence, power, and a perceived lack of hope:

> ... with more and more violence exacted on Gaza, patients reasonably ask: how can we be safe? Where can we go? When will the next war be? You have to try to find the areas in their lives they can control, and you can help with things like improving communication within the family unit.

Hassan, poignantly, equates his work to life in prison:

> Sometimes it's out of their power: it's like for a prisoner. How can he use the period of his confinement in a positive way?[12]

The expression, Gaza is a 'prison camp' or 'open-air-prison' – taken to its logical conclusion – forces us to confront Hasan's view of his patients and himself as prisoners. Other studies, authored by Eyad and others, have revealed how Palestinians described themselves or their futures as broken or destroyed. In the context of an oppressive political context, they use terms like broken, crushed (muhattam), shaken up (mahzuz), destroyed (mudammar), and exhausted, tired (ta'aban). One woman from East Jerusalem was quoted:

> I always try to think positively and have determination and hope, but day after day I feel that I am losing that. I feel as if I am a different person. I feel that my character has changed. It's true that the Israelis give us good money, but they break our souls and determination.[13]

GCMHP was on the frontline of trying to pioneer treatments relevant to this stark context. They were grappling with the tension between a Western canon of mental health treatment for individuals and a society that is not simply collective but deeply bonded by their political conditions. To confront this, GCMHP was at the heart of discussions about mental health, culture and power. It was the first to organize regular conferences that sought to bring mental health experts, even Israelis, together to discuss critical issues.

Their third international conference, organized in 1997, had a rich set of topics, not limited to: the cross-cultural approach to the rehabilitation of survivors of human rights violations, coping modes of current and ex-prisoners, medical ethics and torture, anthropological approaches to children's rights and strategies for schools to address trauma in their pupils. In addition, an academic board was created, and its role would be to keep GCMHP tapped into ongoing scientific research and inform their treatment plans.

GCMHP was at the forefront of treating Gaza's 'traumatized' people. For the first time, school children were able to talk about their trauma: GCMHP introduced expressive writing, drawing and storytelling. In addition, GCMHP would disseminate knowledge to the community to help them understand flashbacks, lack of concentration, nightmares, and temper tantrums, which would lead to more helpful reactions from the children's teachers and parents.

This was undoubtedly necessary work and continues to help the Gaza community. However, the ongoing nature of occupation has led many to critique the use of Post-Traumatic Stress Disorder (PTSD). PTSD is a Western construct that emerged from the experiences of US soldiers returning from Vietnam. In this light, its relevance to the Palestinian context was questioned. Prominent Palestinian psychiatrist Dr Samah Jabr talks about its utility:

> PTSD better describes the experiences of an American soldier who goes to Iraq to bomb and go back to the safety of the United States. He's having nightmares and fears related to the battlefield and his fears are imaginary. Whereas for a Palestinian in Gaza whose home was bombarded, the threat of having another bombardment is a very real one. It's not imaginary. There is no 'post' because the trauma is repetitive and ongoing and continuous. I think we need to be authentic about our experiences and not to try to impose on ourselves experiences that are not ours.[14]

Derek Summerfield, a psychiatrist originally from South Africa but working in London (also a friend of Eyad), contributed to the discussions. He wrote prolifically and fiercely against the use of PTSD as a construct. He considered PTSD to be a post-colonial tool; one which the West would deploy to pathologize and medicalize a normal human reaction to war and violence:

> ...pseudo-scientific pathologizing of people affected by war ... the medicalization of their situation diminishes the importance of work and the rebuilding of social networks ... the broken social world is the lot of the asylum seeker.[15]

These critiques combined offer the space to consider how mental health treatment could be carried out in Gaza. It's not a question of 'should there be mental health treatment?', but rather a question of power and who wields it. It's about not ignoring the voices of Palestinians and instead centering the community, their experiences, and political reality. To not do so risks arrogantly undermining vital coping methods: ones that can provide agency, comfort, and dignity. Eyad knew this approach was essential, and it dovetailed with his intuitive understanding of whence sources of healing came. And as Samah Jabr so profoundly and eloquently states: '*Resilience is the norm; pathology is the exception*'.

The work of GCMHP energized those working in Gaza, mental health researchers and activists from all around the world. As a teenager, I visited Gaza in the 1990s and went to see Eyad at the GCMHP. His office was this big five-storey building right on the beach. Eyad's office had a beautiful view of the

Mediterranean. He liked to start his day with a jog, and some sit-ups, on the beach, followed by office work and meetings.

At this time, Eyad was at the peak of his professional career. He was leading a pioneering NGO, travelling the world, and hosting political salons by night. During the '90s, Eyad spoke at many packed-out halls in the US. He also appeared more frequently in the US media landscape. The pre-eminent NY Times columnist, Anthony Lewis, had written two articles about Eyad, which for the time was unprecedented. Such was his growing public prominence that in 1997, the US-based organization Physicians for Human Rights awarded Eyad their first-ever Human Rights Award, alongside US Senator Patrick Leahy, at its 10th Anniversary gala celebration. Eyad, with the help of supporters in the US such as Nancy Murray, had made substantial inroads into the US public discourse.

The 1990s Gaza was a politically hopeful period. Combined with the hub of energy that GCMHP had become and Eyad's international work, Eyad was surrounded by his beloved family and was not short of warmth, belonging, good company, and lovingly cooked food — in a typical Palestinian way. These were some of the happiest and most productive times for Eyad. He would later lament how sad and lonely he became in Gaza as more and more families left searching for safety and security. It is a testimony to Eyad's sense of purpose and character that he chose to stay in Gaza amidst increasing violence and loss.

Notes

1. Henley, D & Pelling, H 2014, *Eyad El Sarraj: A friend and colleague*, Unpublished
2. Independent Evaluation Group, 2010, *The World Bank Group in the West Bank and Gaza, 2001-2009, Evaluation of the World Bank Group Program*. World Bank https://documents1.worldbank.org/curated/en/144151467998201026/pdf/100011-PUB-P108234-WestBankGaza-CPE-Box393217B-PUBLIC.pdf
3. Wildeman, J & Tartir, A, 2013, 'Can Oslo's Failed Aid Model Be Laid to Rest?' *Al Shabaka*, September 18th
4. Thabet, A, 1999, Visit to the GCMHP training in child mental health, Psychiatric Bulletin,(23) 300-302
5. Aaron, P 2016, 'The Pathological Optimist: One Man's Vision for Palestinian Well-Being', *Journal of Palestine Studies*, V45(2)
6. Friedman, L 2013, *The Lives of Erich Fromm: Love's Prophet*. Columbia University Press, US
7. Lambert, MJ, & Barley, DE 2001, Research summary on the therapeutic relationship and psychotherapy outcome. *Psychotherapy: Theory, Research, Practice, Training*, 38(4), pp.357–361.

8. Aaron, P 2016, 'The Pathological Optimist: One Man's Vision for Palestinian Well-Being', *Journal of Palestine Studies,* V45(2)
9. Filiu, J 2014, *Gaza: A History*, Hurst & Company, London, pp209
10. Henley, D & Pelling, H 2014, *Eyad El Sarraj: A friend and Colleague,* Unpublished
11. National Public Radio (NPR) 2001, 'Fresh Air Archive: Interviews with Terry Gross' 2021. Ruchama Marton'. <https://freshairarchive.org/segments/eyad-el-sarraj> [Accessed 1 October 2021]
12. Dr Hassan Ziada, interview with Tom Hill, 2015
13. Barber, B et al 2016, 'Whither the "Children of the Stone"? An Entire Life under Occupation', *Journal of Palestine Studies*, V45(2)
14. Bland, J. 2017, Profile: Derek Summerfield – politics and psychiatry. *BJ Psych Bull*, Oct; 41(5): 294–296
15. https://www.ncbi.nlm.nih.gov/pmc/articles/PMC5623890/

9. 'IF YOU HAVE THE GUN, YOU HAVE THE RIGHTS'

On September 13, 1993, Arafat signed the Oslo Accords. Arafat had invited Eyad to be part of the Camp David talks. However, despite the careful work of others at Camp David, it was in Oslo that the substantive negotiations took place. The eventual deal itself was widely criticized. Prominent Palestinians such as Edward Said thought the agreement undermined the progress of the *Intifada* and gave away too many concessions. Moreover, the deal would force Israel into ending neither the violence nor the occupation.[1] Eyad was photographed on the day of Oslo waving a Palestinian flag, sitting triumphantly on his friends' shoulders.

With hope and fear in the air, the material reality of the peace process became evident. The Palestinian Authority (PA) establishment was a significant development of Palestinian self-rule. It was supposed to be a 'temporary' institution with limited powers. However, the PA still exists today. The PA struggled to be all things to all people and was described as 'totalitarian...single-party rule, with no accountability.'[2] Eyad was especially upset at what he saw as Arafat bringing tribal loyalty into governance. Eyad observed that Arafat had allowed his security forces to penetrate the tribe, and in return, the tribe penetrated the security forces. For Eyad, this raised serious questions about ensuring the rule of law, fundamental human rights, and transparency.

In this context, one new instrument that would be an informal check on the PA's power was the Palestinian Independent Commission for Citizens' Rights (PICCR). Eyad was invited to be its Commissioner-General. His status as an independent and trusted local figure made him a good choice. In addition to the PICCR, local human rights groups were proliferating. These groups called out violations of human rights by Israel and by the PA. However, there was an unwritten rule that you did not personally criticize Arafat. Eyad broke this rule. In an interview Eyad gave to the *New York Times*, that appeared on May 6th, 1996, Eyad said:

> There is an overwhelming sense of fear. The regime is corrupt, dictatorial, oppressive. There are so many arbitrary arrests now, without charge, without reason. The Authority has nine security organizations, each with its own detention center. And people are systematically tortured.[3]

Eyad had upset a thin-skinned Arafat and dismayed a political culture that didn't want their 'dirty laundry' to be aired in public. As a result, he was arrested and jailed for nine days and held without charge.

Eyad was released after an intense international campaign. In a press conference with the AP on May 27th, 1996, Eyad explained his arrest:

> During my time of detention somebody told me that President Arafat personally is feeling hurt by the quotation that was saying that I was comparing freedom between now and the time of the Israeli occupation.
>
> I still insist that there are certain areas but particularly in areas of human rights that need serious attention. There are arrests, there are tortures in Palestinian prisons, and we have to continue to do everything possible to stop all this to make the security machinery abide by the law. [4]

Eyad was furious with the PA's development into an undemocratic, unaccountable, and violent body. He felt a deep obligation to speak out. A friend and colleague spoke about the arrest:

> The display of cruelty evoked in him an immediate and visceral response. It was intolerable. He never lost this capacity for outrage; he never tried to explain it away. This was his fundamental stance. This was really part of his character: an identification with those who are hurt and dispossessed. He could never remain silent: an almost visceral, physical reaction to injustice [5]

Eyad was released from jail, but confusion over his release emerged. The ICJ reported:

> Speaking at Oxford University last week, Mr. Arafat said that he ordered the release of Dr. Sarraj after he had sent him an apology and a retraction. However, Dr. Sarraj wrote to Mr. Arafat expressing his surprise over the statement and said he had only apologized for the personal pain the newspaper interview may have caused Mr. Arafat and that he stood by the facts and statements he made. [6]

According to the Associated Press, the police made Eyad sign a document promising to respect Palestinian laws. But Eyad said he had added a clause, in his own handwriting, saying he had the right to express his opinions to the media.[7]

Eyad believed that freedom of expression was essential for Palestinian society's healthy growth and functioning. He refused to accept that just because you have the gun, you have the rights. Rights were for everyone. Eyad's refusal to apologize. His guile in inserting the clause was courageous. He knew it would only exacerbate the matter. He was then rearrested. The ICJ reported:

Dr. Sarraj was arrested at his home at 12:30 a.m. Monday, 10 June 1996, by Palestinian Criminal Police without a proper legal warrant and held at the police headquarters in Gaza. On Tuesday, the police searched the Gaza Community Mental Health Centre, confiscated computer diskettes and documents, and ordered the office of Dr. Sarraj closed until the end of the investigation. On Wednesday, in a note received by the PICCR, Dr. Sarraj reportedly wrote:

> I was beaten... I feel that my life is in danger. Rescue me... the situation is grave.
>
> Dr. Sarraj was formally charged and not allowed to confer with his attorneys until 3:30 p.m., Thursday 13 June, in violation of Palestinian Penal Law. Dr. Sarraj's attorneys have stated that he was 'in very poor condition, both physically and mentally'.[8]

Eyad had been arrested twice on false charges. In one of the most ludicrous charges, they had claimed to have found cannabis in his desk. Eyad once told me this wasn't true with typical Arabic dark humour: 'My desk had no drawers!'. Eyad was eventually released. At the time, Eyad's niece was married to Arafat's economic tzar. Many believed that his family's close ties to Arafat had made his release inevitable. However, Eyad was deeply grateful for the outpouring of international support, which he believed also contributed to his release. This event demonstrated to the world Eyad's importance in the fight for human rights, and in 1998 he would go on to be awarded the Martin Ennals Award for Human Rights Defenders.

During this period, the head of Preventive Security in Gaza was Mohammed Dahlan. In an interview, Dahlan explained how he oversaw the arrests of Palestinians in Gaza, many of whom were in Hamas, on the orders of Arafat. He complained of the emotional anguish and 'psychological difficulty' it caused him to arrest his own 'friends'.[9] Eyad admitted that the worst part of the event was that Palestinians carried out the violence on him.[10] The bad blood and animosity that the divisions were causing, coupled with the trauma of torturing your own people, would leave more scars on Palestinian society.

During his time in prison, Eyad made unexpected friends: Fatah had been arresting members of Hamas, and Eyad was now side by side with them. He described their kindness towards him, how they protected him, and how they had long conversations about politics and human rights. After these experiences in prison, Eyad was motivated to try to change things for the better. One thing he tried to do was to instil a culture of human rights into the security forces. He didn't want it to be seen as a purely Western idea but rather a basic human need. He established a human rights training program for prison officers and discovered the officers coming to his training were broadly receptive. In addition, he tied human rights to mental health to demonstrate the link between violence and the impact not just on the body but on the mind.

According to many, it was a very successful and clever way of overcoming resistance to new ideas. However, In Lori Allen's: *The Rise and Fall of Human Rights: Cynicism and Politics in Palestine*, she notes that the broader 'human rights industry', not 'human rights', has led to increased cynicism amongst local Palestinians. Questions remain over exactly how much things have changed. Indeed, the gap between reality and 'human rights discourse' has led many to view human rights organizations as donor-driven 'shops', organizations that – to some – appear to only benefit the staff and its directors.[11]

Despite this valid critique, at an interpersonal level, the experience of Eyad's arrest was profoundly affecting and consequential. Eyad's colleagues describe him, not long after, falling into an – understandable – depression. Yet when Eyad reflected on his time in prison, he also saw positives. His relationships with Hamas prisoners showed the local community that he was a true independent. He said his time in prison helped him win the community's respect.

A colleague of Eyad's retells a story from the time:

> While Eyad was in jail, one political prisoner's wife came with excellent food she'd cooked, which he invited Eyad to share. When Eyad left jail, he told me to deduct $200 from his salary every month and send it to the prisoner without telling them it was from him. I did this for a year and a half. One day the prisoner found me and insisted on knowing who the donation was from. When I had to tell him, he went to Eyad's home crying with gratitude, to ask him why he'd done this. Eyad told him, like he told everyone: If someone helps you, you should help them back more than they helped you.[12]

The Second *Intifada*

The peace talks, on which Arafat had placed all his political capital, were not going well. It left Arafat politically weak, and his clampdown on those carrying out resistance made him look even weaker. In 2000 Ariel Sharon visited Al Aqsa, a holy site in Jerusalem, and this incendiary act sparked off what became known as the Second *Intifada*. The Second *Intifada* became synonymous with the use of suicide bombings. These were carried out by Palestinian factions such as Hamas and the PFLP. It was estimated that approximately 151 were carried out in Israel.[13]

The suicide bombings in Israel were devastating in terms of the loss of Israeli civilians and served no reasonable Palestinian strategic goal. According to Ruchama Marton, the Israeli psychotherapist, the violence also scared Israelis. As a society, she said, they had never expected or been prepared for such violence, insecurity, or fear.[14] How would Israel react? How would their historical trauma impact their collective psyche and reaction? In the years to come, no one was quite prepared for the level of violence of which Gaza residents would be on the receiving end.

Eyad gave serious thought to the new phenomenon of suicide bombing.[15] He felt deeply that violence was not the answer, especially as he knew that these suicide bombings were portraying Palestinians as fanatical monsters. However, he also knew that feelings of humiliation, which Palestinians had felt for decades, needed an outlet. Nothing human was alien to my father. Under difficult conditions, he understood and empathized with the most destructive of human tendencies.

Many often saw the Second *Intifada* as hijacked by Palestinian factions, as opposed to the first, which was seen as more grassroots and organic.[16] This factional problem and divisions in Palestine had been exacerbated by Oslo. Paradoxically, Oslo left Palestinians doing the security work for Israel: PA police were protecting settlers from angry Palestinian demonstrators. It caused public anger and allowed other political groups to occupy the political space abandoned by the PLO and Fatah. Hamas filled this political space and continued its resistance, leading to further Israeli reprisals.

In Gaza, in 1997, Israel sealed off the Strip, prevented fishing boats from going to the sea, and suspended the transfer of tax revenues from Israel to the PA (a vital source of income). Israel had total control of Gaza. From the First *Intifada*, it had essentially used Gaza as a source of cheap labour and flooded Gaza with its own goods. One of the consequences of Oslo was a shift away from this strategy. Israel now sought to restrict movements in and out of Gaza. The chipping away at Gaza's freedoms would only worsen after Hamas' election victory in 2006. But this event highlights that Israel's policy of control over Gaza long precedes the current 'blockade' on Gaza.

Eyad found the Palestinian-on-Palestinian violence devastating, watching his community being ripped apart. However, he also witnessed some unexpected effects, or what he called '*identification with the aggressor*' during his time in jail:

> One day during my last detention I overheard a Palestinian officer interrogating a Palestinian man. He was calmly asking questions, but there were no answers. Gradually, the interrogator's voice rose to a shout. Suddenly, he was screaming: but in Hebrew. I was stunned. That was a graphic illustration of the powerful psychological process of identification with the aggressor. In simple terms, the Palestinian officer who was once a helpless victim in Israeli prison was now assuming the position of power, which in his deepest mind was symbolized by the Israeli officer.[17]

Eyad could see how the fraternal violence, in the context of Israel's occupation, was chipping away at the community's foundations. Eyad was entering a post 9-11 world filled with more violence and division, one that would push him to his limits.

'Gaza, A Dangerous Place!'

In 2003 I visited Gaza and learned that as I had a Gaza ID, I would not be able to leave or enter Palestine without prior permission from Israel: I was effectively stuck in Gaza. During this period, Israel was targeting Hamas leaders such as Rantissi and Sheikh Yassin. It was, of course, Rantissi who had been witness to Israel's rounding up and massacring of Gazans decades earlier. While I was in Gaza, Israel used gunships to target Dr Rantissi. However, they didn't kill Rantissi; instead, they killed his security guard and a passer-by and injured at least 20 civilians.[18] During this attack, I was out buying a suit to attend my cousin's wedding. Eyad had heard the noise from home and called us immediately.

Samir spoke to Eyad and reassured him we were OK. However, we pulled up behind Sheikh Yassin's car on our drive back from the tailor's. He was Hamas's spiritual leader. Fearing that Yassin was an Israeli target, Samir, in his wisdom, decided to take another route. Samir was right: one year later, March 22nd, 2004, Yassin was assassinated in his car by an Israeli Apache helicopter.[19]

Israel was mounting more and more violent attacks on Gaza. They would use F-16s to hit their targets. I remember being in Gaza during that time but not grasping the broader political context. It was a tense period, and Eyad wrote an article, called *'Gaza, a Dangerous Place'*, which detailed one of our experiences:

> Wasseem was glued to the television screen, following the streams of blood in horror. At night we heard people shouting and pointing to the sky. Wasseem and I looked up and we started counting Israeli jets. Among the clouds there were more than fifteen. I had a sinking feeling that Israelis are going to destroy us with their massive power. I was terrified. When I looked up again there were no jets, only stars. I realized then that it was the moving clouds that gave us the illusion of so many Israeli jets. Wasseem and I confessed that we were affected by the communal hysteria and stress.[20]

He ends the piece:

> Yet I'm clinging to the hope that the day in which Israel will be liberated from fear, from racism and from military extremists will come. I'm hopeful that Palestine will be liberated from the humiliation and inhumanity of

military occupation. I am hopeful that our children in Israel and in Palestine will live in peace and in dignity. The day will come when Wasseem will be able to travel as a free man. [21]

Elections

The following year, in 2005, I returned to Gaza. My university thesis was on Hamas. I wanted to interview some of its members. The first interview was with Dr Mahmoud Zahar. Zahar, a physician and a leading figure in Hamas, had also worked with Eyad to champion the rights of Palestinian doctors. Eyad had arranged the interview, and I remember how angry he was that we were running late. He hated not being punctual and was loath to let people down. It showed a level of respect he had for others. It's how he conducted himself, and to me, that spoke profoundly of the level of respect he showed to others.

Zahar was joking with us that he couldn't understand my mumbling, eventually asking my father if I was Scottish! After we finished talking, Zahar wanted to take us on a tour of his small home. We went upstairs, and he showed me a series of holes in the walls of one of his bedrooms. These were the ruinous remains from an Israeli Apache helicopter sent to assassinate him.[22] He survived; his young son was killed. Whatever you think of the politics and strategy, this was yet another story of how the cycle of generational violence only leaves more wounds and ultimately leads to more violence. 'Collateral damage' is never *only* collateral damage.

In the period between 2001 and 2005, the security situation in Gaza had been deteriorating. Arafat installed his brother as head of security but his track record of corruption only inflamed tensions.[23] By all accounts, the PA were in disarray in Gaza. Hamas capitalized and were able to embarrass the PA's security forces. Hamas kidnapped Gaza's police chief and paraded him through the streets in one notable event. The situation in Gaza was described as anarchy. In 2004, adding to the chaos, Arafat passed away. The PA's leader was no more, and his powers were undemocratically transferred to Mahmoud Abbas. After a single election in 2005, Abbas remains in power 16 years later.

As the security context worsened, Sharon declared: 'There will be no Jews in Gaza.' Not long afterwards, I left Gaza, Israel embarked on unilaterally withdrawing from Gaza and dismantling settlements there.[24] By 2005, Israel had withdrawn from Gaza – leaving a total security vacuum. Israel's decision to leave Gaza has been described as 'controlled abandonment'.[25] It's a strategy that allows Israel, once totally dominant, to go, not provide any alternate ways for Gaza to flourish and leave the donor community to foot the human cost. Amidst this security collapse and new reality, there was an effort to conduct democratic elections for the Palestinian Legislative Council (PLC). Eyad, after some encouragement, had decided to stand, but wanted the elections postponed:

> ... how can you proceed with democratic elections? The security forces are not in control. In fact, rather they are the root of the problem. [26]

He accused the militants of damaging the Palestinian cause and scaring away foreigners and aid groups who no longer felt safe in Gaza. For example, the UN bar, where foreigners would spend time, had been blown up. Nevertheless, Eyad still ran for office. He had been encouraged to run as a candidate and ran under a new party called the National Coalition for Justice and Democracy, also known as Wa'ad. Jaber Wishah commented on the reasons for running that year:

> In 2006 we ran in the elections believing we had a narrow chance to make a difference: to raise our voice, to encourage others to believe our principles were worth standing behind: that Eyad's principles were the right of every Palestinian as citizen. We were eager to have elections as the main tool for smooth transfer of power, to pioneer a new, nonviolent political culture in the Arab world. I blame the international community for not standing by the results of the best election occupation could deliver. [27]

In a surprise to everyone, Hamas took 74 of the 132 seats, gaining a majority in the PLC. Immediately the US demanded that Hamas: 1) commit to non-violence; 2) recognize Israel; and 3) respect all previous peace agreements. Further to these demands, Israel prevented Hamas figures from travelling to the West Bank and attending their own PLC sessions. Hamas attempted to form a unity government with the PLO, but an agreement could not be reached. Hamas had won the national elections but were confined to Gaza.[28] The West funded the PA, but now the West refused to pay because of Hamas' win. This meant that 37% of Gaza's civil servants were no longer being paid. Gaza was plunged into crisis. In November 2006, Eyad wrote:

> Hamas's rise to power was well deserved and democratic. It is tragic that Hamas was not ready for this dramatic chance, and it is tragic Hamas was never given a fair chance to govern. After months of pressure and conspiracy, Hamas is yielding to the calls of the community. Hamas should be encouraged and be engaged on all levels, and all conspiracies must stop. A truly democratic culture based on the rule of law is one of the keys to peace.
>
> Fatah and Hamas need to stand behind the leadership of Abbas, who can help the nation and the region because of his unique stature, position and the worldwide respect for his leadership, which is based on his strategic vision of peace-making.

It is time for action. Therefore, I call upon all peace activists to grasp whatever is left of the scattered hopes for peace. Human life is precious and it is our divine duty to protect it. Returning to Gaza and 'normal' life, I am determined to devote the rest of my life to the cause of peace. Peace is freedom. Peace is dignity. Peace is life. [29]

Notes

1. Said, E 1993, The morning after, *London Review of Books*, Vol. 15 No. 20 · October 21st
2. Al Jazeera 2009, 'PLO, History of a Revolution: Intifada',< https://www.aljazeera.com/program/plo-history-of-a-revolution/2009/8/16/plo-history-of-a-revolution-intifada>
3. Greenberg, J 1996, Palestinians in Gaza Arrest Rights Activist, New York Times, May 20th
4. Associated Press 2015, "Gaza Strip: Palestinian Activist Eyad Saraj Released From Jail", YouTube, uploaded by AP, July 21s, https://www.youtube.com/watch?v=RtpHfS3fA1c
5. Husam al-Nono, interview with Paul Aaron, 2015
6. ICJ, 1996, Jurists concerned by arrest of Palestinian Human Rights Commissioner, June<https://www.icj.org/jurists-concerned-by-arrest-of-palestinian-human-rights-commissioner/>
7. Ibid
8. Ibid
9. Neslen, A 2011, *In Your Eyes a Sandstorm. Ways of Being Palestinian*, University of California Press, US, pp170
10. BBC 1997, 'Hard Talk, 'Tim Sebastian interview Dr Eyad Sarraj'
11. Allen, L The Rise and Fall of Human Rights: Cynicism and Politics in Occupied Palestine, Stanford, 2013 pp4
12. Yousef Ghazali, interview with Tom Hill, 2015
13. Benmelech, E 2007, 'Attack Assignments in Terror Organisations and The Productivity of Suicide Bombers', Harvard University and NBER
14. National Public Radio (NPR) 2001, 'Fresh Air Archive: Interviews with Terry Gross' 2021. Ruchama Marton'.<https://freshairarchive.org/segments/eyad-el-sarraj> [Accessed 1 October 2021].
15. El-Sarraj, E, 2002, Suicide Bombers: Dignity, Despair, and the Need for Hope, *Journal of Palestine Studies*, June 1, pp.71–76
16. Khalidi, R 2020, *The Hundred Years' War on Palestine: A History of Settler Colonialism and Resistance, 1917–2017*, Metropolitan Books, New York, pp 175

17. Aaron, P 2016, 'The Pathological Optimist: One Man's Vision for Palestinian Well-Being', Journal of Palestine Studies, V45(2)
18. Filiu, J 2014, *Gaza: A History*, Hurst & Company, London, pp268
19. Hirst, D 2004, 'Sheikh Ahmed Yassin', *The Guardian*, March 22nd https://www.theguardian.com/gall/0,8542,1175396,00.html
20. Sarraj, E 2003, 'GAZA, A Dangerous Place!', Miftah, 13th June <http://www.miftah.org/Display.cfm?DocId=2159&CategoryId=20>
21. Ibid
22. MacAskill, E 2004, 'Leadership may have passed to last founding member left alive', The Guardian, 20th April
23. Filiu, J 2014, *Gaza: A History*, Hurst & Company, London, pp274
24. McGreal, C 2004, 'Sharon plan to move Jewish settlers out of Gaza', *The Guardian*, 3rd February
25. Souri, H 2016, *Gaza as Metaphor*, Hurst and Company, London, pp187
26. Silver, E 2006, 'Anarchy imperils Gaza elections as gunmen seize peace activist', The Independent, 2nd January
27. Jaber Wishah. interview with Tom Hill, May 2015
28. Filiu, J 2014, *Gaza: A History*, Hurst & Company, London, pp305
29. Sarraj, E 2006, 'The campaign that should never stop', Open Democracy, 13 November https://www.opendemocracy.net/en/gaza_campaign_4091jsp/

10. WAR ON GAZA

Israel is pleased to see Hamas take control of Gaza, which will permit us to treat it as a hostile territory.
— Amos Yadlin, Head of Israeli Military Intelligence, 2007

Eyad had bought a small boat in 2005, and one of his great pleasures was taking it out onto the Mediterranean Sea. He would sail out with a few friends and try to catch fish, crab, and shrimp. Anything they caught, they would grill on board for a delicious lunch. I remember seeing how much joy and calmness it brought him. In Gaza, respite is hard to come by. For Eyad going out on the boat, the only boat in Gaza fitted with a toilet, looking out on the horizon, dreaming, hoping, laughing, all this was his privileged sanctuary. But these comforts could not overcome the misery inflicted on Eyad by what became known as the 'blockade' on Gaza.

Deeming it a terrorist enclave, and not part of the 'legitimate' Palestinian Authority, Hamas's 'takeover' of the Gaza Strip allowed Israel to administer a harsh blockade on Gaza. In 2006, as Israel's blockade worsened, Eyad's willingness to try to engage in peace led him and a small delegation to Washington DC. They would meet with President Bush's deputy national security advisor, Elliott Abrams. During the meeting, which took place in Abram's office, they implored him/the administration to consider engagement with Hamas rather than confrontation. But, to their dismay, Abrams made it clear to Eyad that Hamas would be pushed out at any cost. Eyad would later learn that Abrams had been tasked with provoking a civil war between Fatah and Hamas, a decision that would have catastrophic consequences. Reflecting on the internecine violence, Eyad wrote:

> In the savage factional war that lasted for less than a week, Gaza witnessed a wave of brutal atrocities that shocked us all to the core. There were cases of people being thrown from high buildings, wounded people killed in hospital, maimed bodies and scores of tortured victims on both sides.
>
> It is clear that a state of chronic toxicity permeates our society, the accumulation of years of trauma. The Nakba—the uprooting in 1948—the living in refugee camps, the violent abuses and torture by the Israeli army of occupation, the chronic divisions, the lack of leadership, the loss of hope, all have contributed to our tragic, and traumatic situation.[1]

The civil war ended with Hamas keeping hold of Gaza and Fatah retreating to the West Bank. However, with only Hamas in Gaza, the blockade on The Strip was ratcheted up. In December 2008, in the *LA Times*, Eyad wrote very powerfully about the impact of the blockade, which I think is worth sharing in full:

> The advanced medical treatment I need is not available here. But although it is readily available just up the coast in nearby Tel Aviv, I was not allowed to visit my doctor there without permission from the Israelis, who still control our borders and, as the occupying power, remain responsible for the welfare of our civilian population.
>
> In the end, I waited three months for a medical permit to travel to treat my multiple myeloma. My requests were denied repeatedly until an Israeli friend who teaches at Tel Aviv University intervened and helped me secure a one-day permit. That there are still Israelis willing to promote the rights of Palestinians provides me with what little hope I have these days. The majority of Palestinians want only to live with peace and equality, accepting Israelis as our neighbors but not as our superiors or as our jailers
>
> .The situation in Gaza got worse early last month when Israel tightened its blockade of Gaza. Our food, fuel and medical supplies have been severely limited. The blockade has ruined our economy and reduced many among us to a level of economic desperation that has alarmed United Nations officials.
>
> Rather than turn Gazans against Hamas, the blockade's effect has been a humanitarian catastrophe that alienates Gazans young and old from both Israel and the West. Even I, a practicing psychiatrist for decades and a long-time advocate of coexistence between Palestinians and Israelis, am having trouble coping with the hardships to which we are subjected.
>
> Travel is crucial to me, not just for medical reasons but for reasons of basic sanity. I long to see dear friends, to see the world again, to breathe fresh air and, most of all, to reassure my senses that there are normal things and normal people outside Gaza's debilitating confines. The last time I left Gaza, before this most recent medical trip, was several months ago, and the time I spent with friends in Ramallah and Jerusalem was rejuvenating. This time, however, I was only granted permission to leave for a day.
>
> At the Erez checkpoint, where I left Gaza along with four other medical patients, Israeli soldiers spoke through loudspeakers and looked down at us through cameras. 'Open your bag', one shouted. When the woman in front of me asked a question, the soldier ordered her to take everything out of her suitcase. She was humiliated as she had to hold even her underwear up to the camera. I was made to walk through the X-ray machine three times, even though I told the soldiers it was dangerous because of my

medical condition. The soldiers seemed intent not only to determine that we were not bombers but to shame us. What good can come of exercising such domineering power over medical patients?

When one of the soldiers approached us, he was grinning and carrying a huge machine gun across his massive body. I thought that he must feel the power of his muscles and his gun as well as my weakness, with my frail body and my obedience to his orders. But the psychiatrist in me could not escape the question, 'Who is frightened?' — because I was not. I was angry, but not afraid.

On my way back to Gaza, I decided to buy some little plants with flowers to bring home. A soldier shouted at me: Flowers are not allowed.[2]

The blockade, which became more severe after Hamas took over in 2007, meant that Gazans could not leave. This was not only a problem in terms of seeing family but also for life-saving medical treatment. Imports and exports were monitored, with many products being banned, such as pasta. Medical supplies were at all-time lows, with hospitals running out of basics such as gauze. The electricity in Gaza was reliant on fuel from outside of Gaza, but this was in short supply, which meant power only lasted for less than four hours a day. The sea that Eyad, and many other Gazans, used for respite was now filling with thousands of tons of sewage. The one free leisure outlet for Gaza's population was no longer viable, but still, many children would swim in these disease-ridden seas.[3] Gaza was deteriorating, leaving the UN to declare that Gaza would be 'unlivable' by 2020.[4] A phrase many Gazans had started to utter was *Makhnogeen* ('we are suffocating').

Eyad's beloved home was changing beyond recognition. The treatment he was receiving for multiple myeloma and the blockade's impact appeared to have robbed him of his many coping resources. To many, he appeared demoralized. His writing in the *LA Times,* lamenting the changes, is even more tragic as he had no idea that Operation Cast Lead was only a matter of days away.

Cast Lead

Operation Cast Lead started on 27 December 2008 and would not end until 18 January 2009. The operation was said to have been timed before Obama took office and as George Bush vacated the Oval Office. This war on Gaza was devastating, resulting in between 1166 and 1417 Palestinian deaths.[5] It was the heaviest attack on Gaza since 1967 and nothing like anything Eyad had experienced.

During this time, he felt an overwhelming sense of fear that he – and many others – had never felt. As Gaza's 'father' and figure of safety, neighbours would rush to his home seeking sanctuary. He described being constantly on the phone trying to help people decide where they should go to feel safe. But, of course, nowhere was safe. Eyad was frightened. Violence had come not just to his area but also to his home.

During the violence, Eyad had housed a foreign activist, Ewa Jasiewicz. Ewa was an activist who helped protect farmers who were being shot at in the border areas. She regularly put her life on the line. During Cast Lead, she volunteered with the emergency ambulance services with her friend Caoimhe. I had arrived in Gaza just after Cast Lead and met with Ewa and Caoimhe at my father's. It was my first time meeting an activist like Ewa. In one of our first conversations, she described a gruesome scene. Ewa and Caoimhe had arrived in the aftermath of an Israeli airstrike. They found a headless body lying in the street. As ambulance volunteers, Caoimhe had carefully picked up the pieces of skull and brain to preserve for the man's burial respectfully.[6]

Cast Lead lasted almost three weeks: it was thought that $1 billion worth of damage was caused. An estimated 4,100 homes were destroyed, and over 20,000 shelters were damaged. According to UNRWA, the UN relief agency, more than 1,000 Palestinian families were still living in temporary tents a year later.[7] Cast Lead shook my father. He told a group of visiting lawyers from the US Guild investigating war crimes:

> I used to be a peace activist – no more. I don't want peace with a country like Israel. This country has proven that it is living outside of the law. It does not respect human rights at all... Israel is using sophisticated methods of targeted killing and psychological abuse... They are not stupid, they are not evil, they are mentally ill and they need psychological treatment. 85% of the Israeli population supported the war and the atrocities in Gaza.'[8]

My father's boat, which had been such a source of comfort, was destroyed by Israel's F16s. Parts of GCMHP's beachside clinic were damaged, and Eyad's small family were traumatized. Eyad, seen as the protective father figure by many, had failed to protect his community and those closest to him. The peacemaker, the self-described 'pathological optimist', who so often took the moral high ground, sounded demoralized, angry, and hopeless.

Notes

1. Sarraj, E 2008, The Grief Counselor of Gaza, The Link, V41(3)
2. Sarraj, E 2008, Catastrophe for Gaza, LA Times December 14th
3. Beaumont, P, 2017, 'The worst it's been': children continue to swim as raw sewage floods Gaza beach', *The Independent*, 31st July

4. Macintyre, D 2019, 'By 2020, the UN said Gaza would be unliveable. Did it turn out that way?', *The Guardian*, December 19th

5. Amnesty International, 2009, *Israel/Gaza: Operation Cast Lead: 22 days of death and destruction*, July 2nd,<https://www.amnesty.org/en/documents/mde15/015/2009/en/>

6. Jasiewicz, E, 2015, 'I saw a man beheaded', *Red Pepper*, 10th December

7. Almisshal, B 2009, 'Politics hamper Gaza reconstruction', *Al Jazeera*, December 27th<https://www.aljazeera.com/news/2009/12/27/politics-hamper-gaza-reconstruction>

8. Jasiewicz, E, 2015, 'I saw a man beheaded', Red Pepper, December 10th

11. A TALENT FOR HOPE

Everything in this world can be robbed and stolen, except one thing. This one thing is the love that emanates from a human being towards a solid commitment to a conviction or cause.
—Ghassan Kanafani

When I arrived in Gaza in 2010, I found a slightly renewed figure. My father had remarried in 2005 to Nirmeen, who worked as a Human Rights Officer at the United Nations. They had one son, Ali, and Eyad lived with Nirmeen, Ali and Nirmeen's children (Nour and Adam) from her first marriage. These changes helped with his renewal: he often thought about the future of Palestine with his youngest son in mind.

Eyad was back to work advocating through international media to 'end the siege on Gaza'. He wrote articles and appeared on TV to describe its effects and implore the world to act. He was also hosting foreign delegations that had begun to visit Gaza to see the impact of Cast Lead. In their effort to document the impact of Cast Lead, the UN conducted a typically thorough investigation. The investigation was led by Judge Richard Goldstone, a South African Jewish jurist. Eyad was an eyewitness, and in the report, he describes how neither side sees the other as a complete human being and how this dehumanization only adds to a state of paranoia. He concluded:

> I wish that the Israelis (…) would start to walk on the road of dealing with the consequences of their own victimization and (…) start dealing with the Palestinian as a human being, a full human being who's equal in rights with the Israeli and also the other way around, the Palestinian must deal with himself, must respect himself and respect his own differences in order to be able to stand before the Israeli also as a full human being with equal rights and obligations. This is the real road for justice and for peace.[1]

Despite Cast Lead's violence and horror, Eyad still used his public platform to draw attention to a belief in universal humanity. While he never admonished or dissuaded others for using violence, he saw no harm in advocating for a common humanity. And in a *Foreign Policy* article, he again reiterated that Obama, who was stifling the Goldstone report's findings, should:

> [Obama should] ...help Israel's leaders to understand that security cannot be achieved by the gun, but only by readiness to accept me, a Palestinian, as an equal human being with equal rights. [2]

Impasse

In the aftermath of Cast Lead, politically things were still at an impasse. Hamas and Fatah were bitterly divided, and the violent fighting between them had created feelings of revenge and hatred. The material reality of their division meant that Hamas was in control of Gaza, and Fatah was in control of the West Bank. This geographical separation caused great pain to divided families, who were also bitterly divided over which faction spoke for Palestinians. Eyad's independence and social capital, which he had built up in society, meant he could help with some of the consequences of this division.

One life and death issue was medical referrals: Patients in Gaza, like Eyad himself, had to go to Israeli hospitals for life-saving treatments. However, because of the division, the government in Ramallah was holding up applications. Eyad worked closely with Mahmoud Daher of the WHO to leverage his decades of connections. He helped form a committee of figures from the UN, Gaza and Ramallah to help ensure patients could get to Israel. According to those involved, the Minister of Health in Ramallah was not letting in vital equipment to Gaza, and Eyad was furious:

> Eyad called Salam Fayad: 'Listen, your minister is depriving Gaza of vital supplies, including dialysis machines, and people are going to die.' He followed up with a letter to Fayad in which he asked him to dismiss the Minister whom he charged with 'committing crimes against the citizens of Gaza'[3]

He hadn't lost any of his passion or sense of justice. Where Eyad could effect change, he tried. His work behind the scenes allowed patients to get the care they needed and saved lives. It was not a job *per se* but something he was morally driven to do. He never gave up fighting against injustice.

Ubuntu

The Gaza that my father loved was slipping away. He often lamented about his feelings of loss. It had, of course, been changing slowly for decades. Cast Lead and the blockade accelerated its decline. The UN's reports outlined severe man-made catastrophes affecting drinking water supplies, sewage infrastructure overload, and 50% unemployment.[4] My father spent most of his time at home, in the garden, or at his favourite restaurant overlooking the sea. One of the things he liked to do was to go to the sea and eat fish in a small shack. It wasn't luxurious, but he loved to sit, grill the fish and look out at the sea. He had no boat, but he still tried to find respite where he could. I think the pain of Gaza's physical deterioration was sometimes too much to bear. Looking out to sea, or at the garden's plants, was in a literal sense a less painful view.

Eyad's decades of work had won him many friends and admirers. In 2010 he received two important awards: the Juan Lopez Ibor Award, presented as part of the World Psychiatric Congress, and the Olaf Palme Award, named after the former socialist Prime Minister of Sweden. The Olaf Palme award was given in light of 'his self-sacrificing and indefatigable struggle for common sense, reconciliation, and peace in a region characterized by violence, occupation, repression and human misery.'[5] I collected these awards on behalf of my father, who at the time was too unwell to travel. We worked on the speeches together, and it was very meaningful to be able to collect them on his behalf. However, part of me wished I was in the audience. From there, I would have been able to watch Eyad give a typically rousing acceptance speech to his beloved friends and colleagues.

Despite not being able to travel, he was still incredibly active and social. In the years I was in Gaza from 2009 to 2012, I saw Eyad meet and communicate with a host of people: Jimmy Carter, Tony Blair, Naomi Klein, Noam Chomsky, Congressmen Keith Ellison, European MPs, and CNN journalists, to name a few. He enjoyed this role immensely. Eyad would hold court comfortably with these guests, telling them passionately and charmingly how they could help and what they must do. But he was encouraging to everyone. It wasn't just 'VIPs' with whom he engaged. He was willing to sit and engage with anyone willing to help. And if he could help, he would. For example, in a memorial to Eyad, a speaker described *Ubuntu*. It's an African philosophy, defined as:

> *I am because we are... the belief in a universal bond of sharing that connects all humanity.*

One such example of *Ubuntu* is Eyad's friends in America: Bob and Gerri. I first met Bob and Gerri in Seattle when I was a teenager. We were on a family vacation in America. Bob and Gerri were hosting us in their home. My father was enjoying the sea air and looked refreshed. I could also see that Gerri was thoughtful of the stress Eyad was under in Gaza and wanted him to relax. It wasn't until 2011 that I would see Bob and Gerri again, but this time in Gaza. I learned that they try to come every year to Gaza: in 2009, they were part of a volunteer delegation, some of whom were surgeons seeing patients. Gerri wrote in a blog:

> This afternoon, Bob and I returned to a northern Gaza area where a dear friend lives. She and her friends particularly like the homemade chocolates that our Kirkland neighbour, Susan, makes and sends with us each time we visit Gaza. I was so happy to be able to give my friend and her family some of this delicious treat again!
>
> She is a nurse, will have a Caesarian birth later this month – her third child in four years. We hope this third Caesarian will go beautifully.[6]

Bob and Gerri still go every year to Gaza. Connections that mean so much to them and their friends in Gaza, the same people who slip away from view as soon as the bombs stop dropping. These relationships are not rooted in a profession or a career, and they will not be 'scaled' up. They don't require an Instagram account or a declaration that you are the founder, co-founder or CEO of an NGO. They are authentic, sustainable, and away from any limelight. Gerri tells me they still go each year to Gaza in honour of Eyad.

Eyad, his home, was also a safe place for foreigners. For example, Kai Wiedenhofer, an award-winning photographer, was documenting the destruction after Cast Lead. He would spend his day photographing Palestinians who had lost limbs through the violence of Cast Lead. It was a powerful piece of work. Kai would visit us each day after a day's shooting. Eyad's home, and his comforting manner, were a space for Kai to unload and try to refresh himself for the next day. Similarly, the journalist Arthur Neslen took refuge at Eyad's home after a man in need of psychiatric care attempted to stab him. Eyad made Arthur feel safe and protected when he needed it most. This was the often unnoticed solidarity work Eyad did.

Despite efforts towards reconciliation, led by Eyad and others, the political divide between Fatah and Hamas appeared unbridgeable. The divide gave Israel further opportunity to continue to bomb and terrorize Gaza. In 2012 I got my first experience of these bombings during 'Operation Pillar of Defence. I wrote about this for *The New Yorker*:

> In our house we have become military experts, specializing in the sounds of Israeli and Palestinian weapons. We can distinguish with ease the sound of Apaches, F-16 missiles, drones, and the Fajr rockets used by Hamas. When Israeli ships shell the coast, it's a distinct and repetitive thud, marked by a one-second delay between the launch and the impact. The F-16s swoop in like they are tearing open the sky, lock onto their target and with devastating precision destroy entire apartment blocks. Drones: in Gaza, they are called zananas, meaning a bee's buzz. They are the incessant, irritating creatures. They are not always the harbingers of destruction; instead they remain omnipresent, like patrolling prison guards. Fajr rockets are absolutely terrifying because they sound like incoming rockets.

You hear them rarely in Gaza City and thus we often confuse them for low-flying F-16s.

It all creates a terrifying soundscape, and at night we lie in our beds hoping that the bombs do not drop on our houses, that glass does not shatter onto our children's beds. Sometimes, we move from room to room in an attempt to feel some sense of safety. The reality is that there is no escape, neither inside the house nor from the confines of Gaza."[7]

I was experiencing my first war, but my half-brother, Ali, had already experienced Cast Lead, as had Eyad. During that time, I remember trying to keep the kids' spirits up. I would make crepes and put on movies for them to watch. I tried to be stoic, but I was terrified. Recently I found an email from my father that he had written to me after the war:

> I am a proud father and thank you for that. Having you with us Wasseem has given us joy and pleasure, but during the war you took in so much and made me so assured and secure. Thank you my son.

The moving message forced me to reflect that I was now a part of generational violence. It started in 1947 when my father was unable to be protected by his father during the *Nakba*. Then my father tried to protect his youngest son Ali during Cast Lead in 2008. And now, in 2012, I am trying to protect my family and my father. But who is protecting me? During this war, I remember my father mainly being bedridden. I wasn't sure if he was confined to his bedroom because of his illness or fear and helplessness. He was human, after all, and Cast Lead had affected him.

I had to leave Gaza in 2012. The violence I had experienced was too much. I was scared, and traumatized even, but I also felt helpless. Aware of the privilege to be able to leave, I said goodbye – like a prisoner leaving jail. Nine years later, I still experience moments where I relive those bombings. This is a symptom of PTSD. Samah Jabr is right to draw attention to the meaning of PTSD. In the context of Gaza, is there ever a 'post'? My friends and family in Gaza are still living through 'trauma'. In addition to my reliving symptoms, I also lashed out verbally at other activists: I felt hopeless, demoralized, and burnt out. Whatever I was feeling, and doing, was, of course, normal. It was not the first time someone heavily involved in Palestinian rights, who perhaps had also experienced violence, had acted, or felt, like this. It is the human cost of the struggle against structural and colonial violence, and it's what the oppressors hope will force us to give up.

In his final months, Eyad still wanted to help. He was still working on a *hudna* from his hospital bed to bring peace to Palestinians and Israelis.[8] He also wanted to start projects for the youth. Heba Hayek, a young translator, described interviewing for Eyad:

...the appointment (...) took place in Dr. Eyad's living room. To my surprise, he was wearing casual clothes and a pair of slippers. His house, however, was exquisitely furnished. A beautiful gramophone laid on the stool at the right side of the entrance. A large, well-organized library attracted my attention. My admiration for reading made me forget for a second the main reason for our visit. I wanted to go through every book in that library.

Once I sat down, all my fear faded away. 'Your C.V. is very interesting,' Dr. Eyad said. 'It's not easy to find a fluent English speaker with a good background in project management. My assistant will contact you in a few days to assign you the first task. No worries. We'll work together on your management background to empower you in your work.

That was it! All the questions I assumed would be in the interview were not asked. Not only that, but he also praised me and reinforced me and my experience, and he wanted to enlarge on it, as if he saw something in me which I couldn't yet see.

Dr. Eyad lit a light of hope inside every desperate person in Gaza. He dreamed of a better future for Palestine and the people here. For me personally, he gave hope at a time when I had nearly none. [9]

My Way

My father was in an Israeli hospital. It was the second time he had been rushed there from Gaza. I was 'lucky' to have received 'special permission' to fly into Israel. This was a unique privilege that my family's connections were able to make possible. So I booked a flight leaving London and noticed that it was a connecting flight via Frankfurt.

The second leg was El Al, Israel's national airline. Once I get to Frankfurt airport, I go to the gate for my connecting flight. I walk up to the gate, and there is an additional layer of security. A man in a suit greets me: 'Shalom,' he says. I am thinking that this is the high point of our relationship, as once he sees my passport, my name, my place of birth, it will all be downhill. And predictably, it is.

I am taken away by two-armed security guards. They are leading me to an elevator that brings me to the lower ground of Frankfurt Airport. There is no reason to go through my hand luggage, frisk me, and ask me more questions about the 'purpose of my visit'. This has been done multiple times already – but this is the Palestinian experience. I return and am sitting at the gate with the passengers who have seen me disappear and then reemerge. I am sitting alone; they are staring at me with a mixture of fear and disgust. But all I am thinking about is getting to the hospital.

More questions in Ben Gurion Airport, more waiting, more calls by disbelieving airport security staff that a British / Palestinian would have 'permission' to fly into Israel: 'Why didn't you fly into Amman?', she asks, implying that this entry point is not for me, that this is not my country, and I should go the other way! Eventually, I leave the airport and head to Ramallah, where my uncle and aunties stay. They have come from Cairo and Kuwait to be with their brother. Eyad is on life support in an Israeli hospital.

The attending Israeli doctor was pleasant to me. He seemed like a warm figure, and he indicated he knew who my dad was. It was strange being around so many Israelis; I had no idea about their politics. Did they hate me? Had they been in the IDF and killed Palestinians? I would get calls from my father's Israeli friends, who were also visiting and talking to the doctors. These connections meant my dad wasn't 'just a Palestinian'; he was a notable Palestinian with Israeli friends. These Israeli friends could talk in the language that the Israeli doctors understood. My dad wasn't 'just a Palestinian', he was a Palestinian with Israeli friends.

Eyad was in the hospital for about a week; he was never awake during that time. I remember my aunties praying by his bedside, and they at times seemed hopeful. To cope, I was repressing a lot of emotions and spending time alone. Later that evening, I received a call from Gerri. I told Gerri the latest news when she said: 'He loved you in his own way'. I struggled to control my emotions and thanked Gerri for her compassion.

Gerri gently encouraged me to talk to my father and ask my family if there was anything they wanted to say to him. I collected a few things to say from my mother and brother, and the next day I sat by my father's hospital bed. I sat there telling him softly that he was loved, we were proud of his achievements, that he would be missed, and that he shouldn't feel guilty for not being around too much. I don't know if he could hear me, but I hoped he could, perhaps even feeling more peace in his final moments.

'I would rather die with dignity than live in fear' – Eyad

The funeral was in Gaza: I had to get there from Ramallah, a fifty-mile journey in total. So I set off with my cousins very early in the morning, which should have allowed plenty of time. However, we were held up so many times, and for so long, without – of course – any explanation, at various Israeli checkpoints, that I never arrived in Gaza in time to attend the funeral. This is a very familiar experience for Palestinians. And, of course, many Palestinians would not even consider trying to attend a funeral that took place either outside of Gaza or the West Bank.

That day Eyad's burial was attended by Palestinian leaders, including Ismail Haniyeh, Gaza's leader and *de facto* Prime Minister, and was covered by local television. I finally arrived in the evening, late, to play the ceremonial role of shaking people's hands. The community had lined up outside Eyad's home in Remal, with some sitting huddled together. I shook the hands of mourners, along with Ali, who, to shake hands, had to stand on a white plastic chair. I recall many people telling me how kind Eyad was. Stories emerged of how he would regularly give whatever he could to desperate families. People would knock on his front door and inevitably receive some Shekels or Dollars. Eyad had spent much of his life aware, personally and clinically, of the potential impact of the loss of a father. His refusal to leave Gaza, his kindness, gentleness, and his willingness to stand up for truth and justice, had offered the community protection, comfort and hope. He had become the father figure that he felt the community needed.

The whole experience of the funeral was alien to me, and at the time, I felt out of place and mind. However, I was grateful to have played these ritualistic roles in hindsight. Seeing the community come out in such numbers reminded me of a story my father had told me. He joked that when attending his own father's funeral, he kissed so many people on their cheeks that day (kissing on both cheeks is an Arab custom) that he had to apply cream later on in the evening to soothe his skin. I didn't use any face cream that evening, but I was deeply moved by the sense of community, solidarity, belonging, and warmth that was on display that evening.

My father's obituary appeared in the *New York Times*, *Al Jazeera*, *The Guardian* and *The British Medical Journal*, and many more. The United Nation's Special Coordinator also gave him a tribute:

> I was deeply saddened by the news that Dr. Eyad El-Sarraj had passed away. I knew him as an exceptional and dedicated personality, working tirelessly to improve the lives especially of his fellow Gazans, and someone who persistently stood on the side of human rights, peace and justice. It is a big loss for the Palestinian people and their friends. But Dr. Sarraj's legacy lives on and through it he stays in our memory. I send my deep condolences to his family and the people of Palestine. [10]

In Boston, a memorial for Eyad was organized by Nancy Murray and the GCMHP foundation (a US charity to support GCMHP). At the memorial, many figures paid tribute to Eyad, including Sara Roy, Noam Chomsky, and the US/Palestinian Psychiatrist Dr Jess Ghannam. Nancy Murray's tribute seemed to sum up Eyad's achievements and character:

> His courage, decency, independence of mind, and vision of a better world made him a beacon of moral conscience and hope for those Israelis seeking

peace with Palestinians and Palestinians struggling with both the occupation and their own ruinous political divisions.

Testimony to Eyad's global prominence, Desmond Tutu, the world-famous South African Anglican bishop, known for his work as an anti-apartheid and human rights activist, made the following remarks:

> The legacy of Dr. Eyad El-Sarraj will continue in the Gaza Strip as long as organizations like the Gaza Community Mental Health Programme exist to help such victims, their staff caring for the psychologically wounded while often enduring similar trauma as those they treat. God is evident in Gaza, evident by the hearts and hands of those who spread God's Grace and Mercy.
> God Bless You.

But it was the words of his dear friends David and Henrik, who had helped with the early days of GCMHP, that moved me the most:

> We knew that Eyad was not doing well and spent a long evening with him. He had worsened appreciably since our last visit, was nearly totally confined to bed and needed much assistance with all daily activities. And yet we had an enjoyable time, going through our history and talking about all the charming, silly, outrageous, and important happenings we had together. We could say things to each other that hadn't, maybe, been expressed previously. Perhaps we sensed that this would be our last time together.
>
> Several days after returning home we checked the Facebook, and there Eyad had posted several communications. There were pictures of us together, one from a walk on the beach, with the words, 'The good old days and the daily walk on the beach', the others from our recent evening together, with a message saying something like, 'Thanks for the evening and for what started in Uppsala 24 years ago.'
>
> We scrolled down a little further to a new message from Eyad, a video with Frank Sinatra, who was singing 'My Way'. Then the tears came. [11]

Notes

1. UN Human Rights Council 2009, 'Human Rights in Palestine and Other Occupied Arab Territories: Report of the United Nations Fact-Finding Mission on the Gaza Conflict', September 25th<https://www2.ohchr.org/english/bodies/hrcouncil/docs/12session/A-HRC-12-48.pdf>

2. Sarraj, E 2010, 'Gaza's Agony', Foreign Policy, January 27th
3. Mahmoud Daher, interview with Tom Hill, 2015
4. Human Rights Watch 2020, 'Israel and Palestine Events of 2019',<https://www.hrw.org/world-report/2020/country-chapters/israel/palestine>
5. Olaf Palme Foundation 2010, 'Eyad Sarraj'<http://www.palmefonden.se/2010-eyad-el-sarraj-2/>
6. Haynes, G 2014, 'Day nine in Gaza: Saying goodbye to friends', Larry Johnson Online, April 12th<http://www.larryjohnsononline.com/?paged=5>
7. El Sarraj, W 2012, 'The Sounds in Gaza City', New Yorker, November 19th
8. Erlich, E 2018, 'Only a Reconciliation Delegation Will Bring About a Cease-fire', *Haaretz*, June 19th
9. Hayek, H, 2021, 'Dr. Eyad El-Sarraj: A light of hope for Gaza', We Are Not Numbers, March 4th
10. UNSCO 2013, 'Statement by UN Special Coordinator Serry on the passing of Eyad El-Sarraj', December 13th<https://www.un.org/unispal/document/auto-insert-195678/>
11. Henley, D & Pelling, H 2014, Eyad El Sarraj: A friend and colleague, Unpublished

12. THE RATIONALITY OF REVOLT

Not everything that is faced can be changed, but nothing can be changed until it is faced.
—James Baldwin

In 2014, Israel launched another attack on Gaza. It lasted seven weeks and fit a familiar pattern of Israel striking Gaza in 'retaliation' for Hamas rocket fire. But the history, when laid bare, shows violence towards Gaza to have been persistent and calculated. Over 2000 Gazans were killed, and 10,000 families were displaced. In one single Israeli airstrike Dr Yasser Abu Jamei, a friend of Eyad's and the new director of the GCMHP, lost 28 relatives, including three pregnant women. I reflected on these events for the *New Yorker*:

> Even now, after the bombing, Yasser tells me that he will try to steer GCMHP on the path that Dr Eyad, as he was invariably called, set. Some observers might call this typical steadfastness, or samoud: a sort of mystical quality often used to describe Palestinians, particularly at times like these. But it doesn't seem honest to speak of steadfastness, really. Rather, it's a question of Yasser and the many other mental-health practitioners who will be so needed in the wake of yet another war, who have no choice but to stay in Gaza and deal with unspeakable tragedies not only in other's lives but in their own, honoring my father's mission as they do so. That's not steadfastness or samoud. That's life.[1]

In a 2016 interview, Yasser detailed some of the GCMHP's work in the aftermath of this violence:

> In the three GCMHP centers across the Gaza Strip, in the last year or so—from August 2014 until July of this year—almost 35 percent of our adult clients have exhibited a major depressive disorder and another 25 percent have post-traumatic stress disorder (PTSD). We believe that the last offensive had the greatest impact not only because of the level of destruction but because of the losses associated with that destruction: loss of people, loss of houses, the sheer scale of the destruction, as well as the desperate lack of employment opportunities. That's why we think that the adults who came into our clinics exhibited more depression than trauma.
>
> With children, the opposite is true. Up to now, some 45 percent of children coming into our community centers have PTSD and another 10 per-

cent suffer from bed-wetting episodes. In the last year, ever since the last offensive, we have been seeing three or four major issues in children: bed-wetting; poor school performance; problems with discipline; and, lastly, night terrors, which are episodes of uncontrolled screaming in the middle of the night when the child continues to scream while asleep and remembers nothing after being woken up."[2]

Eyad, too, would have tried to make sense of the scale of suffering. However, some people say he was spared from seeing more carnage. Thankfully, before the 2014 attack, Nirmeen (Eyad's wife) had already moved Ali, and her small family, to start a new life in Switzerland. But, of course, not everyone was so privileged. Gaza's almost complete deterioration sparked a new phenomenon: Palestinians fleeing Gaza by boat. Gazans hoped that they too could find safety and security elsewhere by paying smugglers. In 2014 tragic stories started to emerge of the perilous attempts to cross the Mediterranean. A boat containing 500 people was rammed by smugglers when the captain refused to move his people onto a smaller boat fearing they would all die from the weight. As a result, at least 200 Palestinians from Gaza drowned, as did the captain. A tragedy reminded me of the loss of life caused by the Struma disaster 72 years earlier.

In 2014, around the time of this latest episode of violence, I was in London. I had been asked to host an event with Mads Gilbert. Mads Gilbert is a Norwegian doctor who treated patients at Shifa during the Israeli bombings. He describes himself as a "political doctor" and a practitioner of "solidarity medicine". He worked 30-hour shifts with Palestinian medics:

> "It's a place of human greatness, suffering and endurance – and an almost incomprehensible mastering of a situation that seems overwhelming, impossible to deal with. Yet they [the medical staff] stand tall, don't reject a single patient, do phenomenal, very complicated surgery with a high level of professionalism".[3]

It was poignant to think that Shifa, the hospital that Eyad fought to work at, where he treated so many patients, remains such a sight of incredible suffering. Yet, the many doctors, nurses, and cleaners, who work and have worked there over the decades are quiet, unsung heroes. They don't have memoirs or awards, but their efforts must not be forgotten.

'The reason that it looks like apartheid is simply because it is apartheid.'

With the election of Trump in 2016, many saw the deterioration of Palestine hastening. Trump's son in law, Jared Kushner, embarked on 'solving the Israel/Palestine problem'. But he only saw a 'conflict' that would be resolved through economic incentives. It was a narrow vision of Israel and Palestine and expectedly led nowhere. Nathan Thrall, a scholar of the peace process, gave the following summation of over 40 years of US-backed and UN-supported, Israeli/Palestinian peace talks:

> Through pressure on the parties, a peaceful partition of Palestine is achievable. But too many insist on sparing Israelis and Palestinians the pain of outside force, so that they may instead continue to be generous with one another in the suffering they inflict.[4]

In reaction to being fenced into Gaza, bombed, and with no serious effort to foster peace, Palestinians in Gaza – once again – attempted to take back their agency, their destiny and organised the 'Great March of Return'. It was a non-violent, grassroots initiative to gather peacefully near the border with Israel. The protests were met – with what some medical observers described as 'calculated maiming' – by Israeli sniper fire.[5] 214 Palestinians, including 46 children, were killed, and over 36,100, including nearly 8,800 children, have been injured. Over 7,000 live ammunition injuries (some 88%) were limb injuries, followed by injuries to the abdomen and pelvis. The 156 of the limb injuries have resulted in amputations (126 lower limb and 30 upper limb). Out of these, at least 94 cases involved secondary amputations due to subsequent bone infections.

During the Trump administration, Gaza continued to be bombed. In 2019, during one of these rounds of bombings, our family home was hit by an Israeli airstrike. I was in London when my wife, Hiba, said she wanted to show me something, warning me that I should be prepared. She put her iPhone in front of me; a series of photos of my father's home was on the screen. One photo showed Eyad's portrait, once hung proudly over the dinner table, lying on the ground, covered in rubble. Another showed a huge gaping hole in the kitchen wall. You could see right through to the outside and past the basketball net that Ali and I used to play with. If I had been in this home or making pancakes in the kitchen, I, or my family, would be severely injured or dead. The target of the bombing, according to Israel, was a Turkish media organisation housed next door. Media organisations have long been targets for Israel, and Israel has not been held accountable for its actions.

I was glad my father was spared more pain: no one deserves this.

In 2021 the Israelis launched another attack on Gaza. This was different to 2014, 2012, and 2009, in that the fuse was lit in Jerusalem. It's not without precedent that actions in Jerusalem spark violence. However, in recent times, Israel's rationale for launching attacks on Gaza had been limited to Hamas' firing of rockets. In 2021, the residents of Sheikh Jarrah, a neighbourhood in East Jerusalem, were being forcibly removed from their homes. Israel captured this part of Palestine in 1967 and, through its courts, claims legal rights over the Palestinian homes. Describing this event as a 'real estate dispute' grossly glosses over a hundred years of violence and occupation.[6] There were Palestinian protests across Gaza, the West Bank and in 'mixed cities' in Israel, leading many to declare this a moment of shared Palestinian solidarity, despite geographical separation.[7]

Israel responded with a brutal crackdown on protests and heavy bombing of Gaza.[8] The violence lasted two weeks: 256 Palestinians died, and many parts of Remal, where my father's home is, were bombed. Hamas, during this violence, had repurposed British colonial munitions, which they had rescued from Gaza's seabed. The resourcefulness and willingness to fight back gave Palestinians a sense of needed dignity. However, the 2021 war was the fourth in 13 years, summed up in a tweet by Jehad Abu Salim:

> "That's it, we will die." [A message Jehad received from his sister in Gaza.] Due to the intensity of the situation.
>
> My sister was 8 during the 2008 war, 12 during the 2012 war, 14 during the 2014 war, 18 during the march of return, and now she's 21 during this."[9]

During this violence, my cousin, Yusra, was in the family home with her uncle, Eyad's brother. Only a year before, Yusra had been studying in London. She enjoyed London and imagined staying. Yusra liked the freedom, the peace, the cafe culture and the opportunities it afforded. Her time in London was cut short due to Covid restrictions. Wanting to see her father and be near her family, she returned to Gaza

It was Eid, and optimistically, nobody expected such violence during these yearly celebrations. Hiba and I messaged her daily, and she sent terrified voice notes over WhatsApp of the sounds of bombs falling. She described depression in the subsequent days. Not long after, she was lucky enough to be able to leave Gaza. She described the experience as the worst of her life. She said she wished her 'Uncle Eyad' had been around. She said he would have made her feel safe and would have understood how to help her with her feelings.

The 2021 war, however, did give renewed optimism to supporters of Palestine. It felt to many that Israel could no longer obfuscate the truth: *"Believe your eyes. Follow your conscience. The reason that it looks like apartheid is simply because it is apartheid"*.9 Human Rights Watch and Israeli human rights groups also described what is happening in Palestine as apartheid.[10] Furthermore, prominent Jewish voices have been making a case for a right to return for Palestinians.[11] These two shifts come about as a result of the failure of the 'Peace Process', the intensity and frequency of violence enacted by Israel, Israel's political shift to the right, and to a lesser extent, the Black Lives Matter movement, which helped emphasise human rights within oppressive systems.

There was a substantial global outpouring, with demonstrations that lasted weeks beyond the end of the violence. Celebrities such as Dua Lipa, Gigi Hadid, John Legend all lent their support to Palestine. Prominent Palestinian activists living in Palestine were also given celebrity status, with *Time Magazine* awarding them a place in their "100 Most Influential" list.[12] While it may sound shallow and superficial, their words and actions will shape and inspire the next generation of Palestinian activists. And *Time Magazine* giving credence to Palestinian resistance marks a significant shift in Western discourse.

A Pew Research Center survey also found that only 40% of US Jewish adults thought the Israeli prime minister provided good leadership, falling to 32% among younger Jews. And only 34% strongly opposed sanctions or other punitive measures against Israel, while 16% said that caring about Israel is "not important" to their Jewish identity.[13] Linked to this shift in opinion and discourse are the efforts of big corporations to refuse to trade in Israel's illegal settlements. The ice-cream company Ben and Jerry's no longer will sell in areas deemed unlawful by international law, underscoring the moral imperative of ethical trading.[14]

In 2001 Nancy Murray and Elaine Hagopian founded the US-based GCMHP foundation. They aimed to help raise funds for the GCMHP, and over the years, Nancy organised for Eyad to speak to audiences in the US. She also organised Eyad's 2014 memorial service in Boston. Nancy and many others have been engaging in tremendous acts of solidarity to raise awareness and much-needed funds for the GCMHP and Palestinians. So, it is heart-warming and encouraging to know that, despite Eyad no longer being with us, in 2021, the GCMHP foundation had its most successful fundraising year ever.

The shifting sands of American Jewish support, Palestinian-led demonstrations inside Palestine, celebrity-led global advocacy, and reframing what is happening in Palestine as Apartheid gives many hope. Despite Israel's immense power, they can't crush solidarity or erase the truth, and in many ways, this is what Eyad was working towards his whole life.

Notes

1. El Sarraj, W 2014, 'Fathers and Sons', New Yorker, July 26th
2. Dawson, B 2016, 'Interview with Dr. Yasser Abu Jamei: The Gaza Community Mental Health Programme' Journal of Palestine Studies, Vol 45(2) Winter,

3. Sherwood, H 2015, 'Doctor Mads Gilbert on working under siege in Gaza's Shifa hospital: 'My camera is my Kalashnikov'', The Guardian, June 23rd

4. Thrall, N 2017, 'Israel-Palestine: the real reason there's still no peace', The Guardian, May 16th

5. UNISPAL, 2020, 'Two Years On: People Injured and Traumatized During the "Great March of Return" are Still Struggling', April 6th

6. Adams, P 2021, 'Jerusalem's Sheikh Jarrah: The land dispute in the eye of a storm', BBC News, May 26th

7. Asi, Y 2021, 'The Sheikh Jarrah Chapter of the Palestinian Nakba', Arab Center Washington DC, May 14th

8. Shakir, O 2021, 'Jerusalem to Gaza, Israeli Authorities Reassert Domination', Human Rights Watch, May 11th

9. Salim, J. [Jehad Abu Salim] 2021, ' That's it, we will die. My sister was 8 during the 2008 war, 12 during the 2012 war, 14 during the 2014 war, 18 during the march of return, and now she's 21 during this. [Tweet]', Twitter, April 13th.<https://twitter.com/jehadabusalim/status/1392902993683501058?lang=en>

10. Malik, N 2021, 'Abandoned by governments, Palestinians rely on the kindness of strangers', *The Guardian*, 24th May

11. Wallace -Wells, B 2021, 'A liberal Zionist's move to the left on the Israeli-Palestinian conflict', *New Yorker*, May 23rd,

12. Time 2021, 'The 100 Most Influential People of 2021: Muna El-Kurd and Mohammed El-Kurd', *Time Magazine*, September 15th<https://time.com/collection/100-most-influential-people-2021/6096098/muna-mohammed-el-kurd/>

13. Nortey, J 2021, 'U.S. Jews have widely differing views on Israel', Pew Research Center, May 21st

14. Malik, N, 2021, 'Corporate activism is too often cynical. In Ben & Jerry's case, it offers hope', *The Guardian*, July 25th

EPILOGUE

It is the task of the ethical thinker to sustain and strengthen the voice of human conscience, to recognize what is good or what is bad for man, regardless of whether it is good or bad for society at a special period of its evolution. He may be the one who 'crieth in the wilderness,' but only if this voice remains alive and uncompromising will the wilderness change into fertile land.[1]
—Erich Fromm

When Israel declared itself a state in 1948, Palestinians could not have imagined that it would lead to over 70 years of continued violence, the loss of so much of their land and the destruction of their communities. This entirely man-made tragedy needed the support of other much more powerful countries: Britain and then the US. These global powers operated in different ways for different reasons. Still, the conclusion was that neither did – or does – enough to stop Israel's incessant efforts to ethnically cleanse Palestinians from their land. The UN has tried to establish moral authority – primarily through its application of international law. Its reports offer a powerful and essential record of war crimes, but its limited power and remit don't benefit Palestinians in the short term.

In the context of this ongoing dispossession and violence, Gaza is an exceptional part of the story. Gaza is home to 2.1 million Palestinians, and it's the largest coherent Palestinian territory. Since 1948 Gaza has been on the receiving end of 12 major military campaigns. The violence that Israel enacts against Gaza is, on the surface, a 'strategic' goal to defeat 'terrorism'. However, a closer reading of history shows that the violence has not stopped and is instead carried out with ruthless rigour.

Israel's massive use of force, and its blockade of Gaza, only create hatred and offers nourishment for political groups who fill the void left from any demonstrable progress towards peace. It is, then, perhaps no surprise that out of this desperation and violence have emerged the political groups and leaders of Palestinian politics. Gaza is where many of the founding leaders of Fatah, the PFLP, and the PLO emerged and is also home to Hamas and Islamic Jihad. Eyad's prescient warning of what comes after the suicide bombers of the Second *Intifada* remains an open-ended question.

Amidst this historic brutality, complex local culture, and international attempts to broker peace, Eyad tried to live a life of purpose in service to his community from his home in Gaza. Through his service, he would involve himself in peace talks, write prolifically to raise awareness of the suffering in Palestine, and try to tend to the wounds of the community.

Work and Legacy

Over the years, efforts toward reconciliation and peace have been a mainstay. While the details and tenor vary, the outcome of their resounding failure has remained largely static. Like many others acting in good faith, Eyad tried to support the process. One critique has been that Palestinians have perhaps been too ready to hope for the 'goodwill' of the British or the US. This acquiescence is often considered counterproductive.[2] It is this which has given succour to a new generation of Palestinian activists who see the peace talks as merely a cover for the continued taking of Palestinian land.

For Eyad, I think he saw it as one of the few tools he had at his disposal. Irrespective of whatever was happening, one had to get people to talk, compromise, and see an alternative path out of violence. But it would be wrong to characterise him as someone only involved in 'talking shops', 'elite led' initiatives and a benefactor of the 'conflict resolution industry'. He also led many grassroots initiatives with activists from across traditional lines, such as the 'breaking the siege of Gaza' campaign or the Physicians for Human Rights.

Eyad's love for his community led him to politics; he was not driven by a self-serving ego and would never have been renumerated for his political activism. His day job was as a psychiatrist, and as Gaza's first psychiatrist, he was in a powerful position to pioneer mental health treatment. Before GCMHP, there was almost no mental health treatment infrastructure in Gaza. Since its establishment in 1992, GCMHP has become one of the most essential organizations in the Gaza Strip. Not just in saving lives but in training generations of future therapists, pushing to destigmatize mental health and for it to be seen as a human right (a groundbreaking link), and healing a community victim to such brutal violence. GCMHP is a proud outcome of Eyad's sense of purpose, creativity, and hard work.

When he wasn't working as a psychiatrist, managing an NGO and trying to reconcile warring parties, Eyad was a storyteller and writer. In a largely pre-social media era, this was even more important in helping to dispel myths about Palestine. Eyad was able to publish and speak in many Western media outlets. His contributions provided opportunities to counter the bias of the Western media. For example, less than 2% of the nearly 2,500 opinion pieces that discussed Palestinians since 1970 were written by Palestinians in the New York Times. In the *Washington Post*, the average was just 1%.[3] Media work, without material improvements to your cause, can feel demoralizing and pointless. Still, his (and others') contribution to culture helped lay the foundations for today's social media activists and campaigners to break down systemic media bias.

Palestinians face Israel's immense military power and violence, backed up by the United States, a multi-billion aid industry that decides how much aid and when Gaza should receive it – and a media that too often overlooks Palestinian voices. Up against these forces, Eyad was, in some ways, a buoy bobbing in rough seas. But with moral courage and purpose, he was able, together with his friends, to navigate the rough waters to achieve his goals and maintain his creative spirit, identity, and dignity.

'How can you be an artist and not reflect the times?' – Nina Simone

Gaza's pain was Eyad's pain. Like an artist, in being so intertwined, so connected, so in love, with Gaza, he fought for it regardless of ideology and often with little regard to the personal cost he would bear. The anchoring of the community, and his belonging to Gaza, were decisive protective factors. There is both peace in the intimacy and meaning he derived from this and sadness from the pain he must have felt from seeing the deterioration continuing all around him. But despite the violence and material deterioration, he remained secure in himself. The comfort and coherency he felt gave rise to a personal sense of assuredness. What then emanated from him made others feel protected, hopeful, and consoled in his company? Many Palestinians referred to him as a father figure, and visiting foreign nationals would return to him, assured that he would greet them with feelings of hope, encouragement, and generosity of spirit.

To sustain his work and sense of purpose, Eyad would have to make sense of what was going on around him. Fundamentally, Eyad saw two collections of humans, each in part reacting to their different – and ongoing – traumas. He keenly observed how paranoia, if left to fester, would only lead to further dehumanization. And he believed that additional violence, enacted in the context of historical trauma, would only lead to worse forms of violence. To combat this, he thought that Israelis and Palestinians needed to understand one another better. In this regard, we may call him a *humanist*, someone who tried to see commonalities across humanity.

Perhaps this tendency to see aspects of ourselves in each other was partially rooted in his early childhood. He learned through his connection to his father's friend that Jews were not 'monsters'. On the contrary, he truly believed that if these collections of humans extended empathy and understanding to one another, something good, something better, would come from it. If only Israel would see me as human, he would often say. His time abroad, and his privilege, all helped to strengthen a core belief that, under the right conditions, we could all act humanely towards one another.

Eyad was operating in a community that was not fortunate to have many of his experiences. His humanistic vision would often put him at odds with the community. A people of whom the majority were refugees living in squalor, with memories (and lived experience) of massacres passed down through the generations. His pleas for a reasoned collective human consciousness were regularly tested. Hope is a talent, and a skill, taking practice and helpful conditions. He admitted that not resorting to violence in the face of violence was a personal struggle.[4] In this context, I don't know how he would have made sense of the ferociousness and length of violence carried out on Gaza in 2014 and 2021.

Hope and Solidarity

I was recently visiting Hebden Bridge, West Yorkshire. It's a tiny market town in the North of England, with a population of 4,500. I was walking through its square and noticed a woman with grey hair holding the flag of Palestine. She was alone. I went over and could see she had a table filled with pamphlets and information on Palestine. We began talking, and she asked me if I was Palestinian. In the middle of writing this book and immersed in knowledge about my father's life, this simple question evoked so much meaning. I was Palestinian, I thought, but where do I begin? I held back my emotions, and we talked some more. As I walked away, I thought to myself how wonderful it was that she came out as often as she could to spread awareness of the situation in Palestine. I thought if Eyad had been there, he would have joked with her, encouraged her, and told her that what she was doing was much needed and appreciated.

Eyad is one of many Palestinians who were born into their historical trauma. Palestinians are many things; they are 'original' Gazans, refugees, intellectuals, resistance fighters, exiled, and each, in their way, is trying to live a life of purpose and dignity under intolerable conditions. What Eyad's life demonstrates is that the struggle is collective. It requires solidarity, community, institution building, and the inspiring of hope in one another. A hope and solidarity that can be aided through authentic and caring relationships. In real life and online, the forging of such relationships built around solidarity and justice is perhaps the most beautiful thing I learned from my father's life. Of course, many may disagree with some of Eyad's politics and ideas. Still, the ability to encourage so many, and inspire, especially in such a long struggle, is an important and necessary talent.

I often wished my father had been more present. But now, seeing how closely his soul was tied to Gaza, how he offered such material and symbolic protection to his community, it seems almost cruel to wish that he had stayed on in London.

I left London, where the ideology of individualism and consumerism is both pervasive and insidious. I had been reading Erich Fromm, the psychoanalyst and humanist, in search of answers and escape. After working and living in Palestine, I have come away seeing that there is a different way of being in the world. Fromm would have understood – if not, prescribed – this, and his writing in many ways led me to Palestine and to Eyad.

> 'My humanity is caught up, and is inextricably bound up, in yours. We belong in a bundle of life. We say: 'A person is a person through other persons.'

Geographically Gaza was said to exist at a crossroads. Perhaps Eyad also existed there. Through his commitment to *Ubuntu*, he tried to keep those of us who passed through and those who lived in Gaza united, inspired, resistant to demoralization and hopeful. And through doing this recreated a melting pot of identities that echoed the Palestine of the 19th Century. One of my last memories of my father was walking into his bedroom in Gaza and seeing him lying in bed singing with his young son Ali. They listened to one of *Baba's* favourite songs: Louis Armstrong's *What a Wonderful World*. It's a song that Ali and I will always have to remember him by. God bless *his* wandering soul.

Notes

1. Friedman, L 2013, *The Lives of Erich Fromm: Love's Prophet*, Columbia University Press, US
2. Khalidi, R 2020, *The Hundred Years' War on Palestine: A History of Settler Colonialism and Resistance, 1917–2017*, Metropolitan Books, New York, pp 53
3. pp 533. Nassar, M, 2020, *972 Magazine*, 'US media talks a lot about Palestinians — just without Palestinians', October 2nd
4. BBC 1997, 'Hard Talk, Tim Sebastian interview Dr Eyad Sarraj'

AFTERWORD BY YASSER ABU JAMEI, DIRECTOR OF THE GCMHP

It's hard to believe that it has been thirty years since the Gaza Community Mental Health Program (GCMHP) was established. Dr Eyad, nor anyone else, could ever have imagined that it could have lasted this long, nor could he have dreamed that it would become such an essential part of the community. GCMHP has transformed how mental health has been discussed and treated in Gaza. Eyad's personal sense of right and wrong, and a keen sense of justice, meant that mental health would become inextricably linked with human rights. Under my stewardship, as the current director of GCMHP, we are trying to follow the path Eyad so carefully laid for us.

'Great idea!' Dr Eyad would often say. These were not empty words. He knew that inspiring the staff of GCMHP was critical to their sense of self-worth. I think he took great pride in trying to nurture our confidence. He was also someone who did not try to keep things to himself, and his instinct was to share what he had with others: everything for everyone. Not to be overlooked was his sense of humour. Eyad always had a story, or joke, to share with us; these moments of joy he brought would become even more critical during difficult times.

One of the many ethical lessons Eyad imprinted on us was his refusal to lose sight of truth and justice. This was his guiding light. We would watch him speak in meetings with great urgency and passion. In private and in public, this sense of needing to act now—or needing to try—whatever we could do to improve life in Gaza never wavered. He wrote prolifically, and his writing in Arabic and English instilled hope in all of us. But the hope he had for a better world was not only through his words but also his deeds. He was willing to take on those in power who acted without accountability; these actions made us trust, respect, and believe in him. 'What can we do', he would say to us, but it was always 'we', him and us, together. He was like a father figure to many of us, and we all took great comfort from his refusal to leave Gaza.

I have tried to follow in Eyad's footsteps, not just in leading GCMHP but also in trying to communicate to the world what is happening in Gaza. Eyad inspired us all when we would see him interviewed on the BBC or see his writing in the *New York Times*. Twenty-three years since Eyad appeared on the BBC's popular show 'Hard Talk', I followed suit and gave my interview. I detailed the harsh reality of life in Gaza and tried to explain the importance of GCMHP's work on the show. It was a critical moment for me, but also a realisation that not only does the struggle for justice continue, but that the next generation must – at some point – take over. In this context, I am glad that Eyad's work and his life have been documented and consolidated in this memoir. Dr Eyad was a visionary, and he gave his life to support mental health and human rights in Palestine. In remembering him, we can also continue to be inspired by his actions. Sadly, Dr Eyad passed away in December 2013, but we all carry his torch and strive to continue his legacy.

www.ingramcontent.com/pod-product-compliance
Lightning Source LLC
Chambersburg PA
CBHW070847160426
43192CB00012B/2337